THE GUERRILLA DIET & LIFESTYLE PROGRAM

FROM EVOLUTION TO HEALTH REVOLUTION

Wage War On Weight and Poor Health and Learn To Thrive In The Modern "Jungle"

BY GALIT GOLDFARB

To my teammates in life and on this journey! We are all in this together!

© Copyright 2015

All rights reserved. No part of this book may be reproduced or transmitted in any form or by any means, electronic or mechanical, including photography, recording, or in any information storage retrieval system without written permission from the author and publisher.

Published by: Predicted Achievement

ISBN-13: 978-96592556-1-0

ISBN-10: 96592255616

Cover design: Liv Gold
Layout and typesetting: Liv Gold
Editor: Marlene Oulton, www.MarleneOulton.com

Printed in the United States of America

Acknowledgements

This book is the product of many minds to whom I am thankful. The people who recorded what they saw, the explorers, researchers, scientists, doctors, archeologists and many more, of which I reviewed their essays, periodicals, research papers and reviews for my doctoral program to find the ideal diet for humans, I am truly grateful for their fine work. Without their hard work, this book would never have been possible.

I am also grateful for all my friends, family members, and clients who have tried and tested this material on their own bodies and have been truly pleased with the results.

I also feel a deep sense of gratitude to:

- My wonderful husband for supporting me on this journey. I could not have succeeded without his help.
- My children who have shown me what life is all about.
- To my parents who gave me the gifts I possess and have been a source of inspiration all along the way.
- To Idan Reich for his integrity as well as his editing and refinement of the original manuscript.
- To Marlene Oulton for creatively editing my writings

And... I thank GOD for giving me this life and this wonderful world to live in.

Table of Contents

THE GUERRILLA DIET & LIFESTYLE PROGRAM

Acknowledgements	3
Table of Contents	5
Introduction	7

SECTION 1 13

Evidence Based Background Behind The Guerrilla Diet and Lifestyle Program - The Best Diet for Human Consumption

Chapter 1 — 15

Why "Dieting" Doesn't Work

Chapter 2 — 19

Why Human Needs are Different From Gorilla Needs Even Though Our Similarities

Chapter 3 — 39

An Evolutionary Perspective on Human Diet and Lifestyle

Chapter 4 — 67

Dietary Requirements: Comparison Between Apes and Humans

Chapter 5 — 89

Human Health – Ancient Times vs. Modern Times

Chapter 6 — 99

The Theory Behind Reducing Meat Products in Your Diet

Chapter 7 — 127

The Theory Behind Removing Milk Products From Your Diet

Chapter 8 — 143

The Science of Epigenetics for the Prevention/Reversal of Disease and Weight Issues

Chapter 9 — 153

Principles of Healthy Sleep

Chapter 10   **165**

Neuroplasticity and The Principles of a Positive Mindset

Chapter 11   **177**

An Evolutionary Approach To Physical Activity Needs

SECTION 2 183

The Guerrilla Diet & Lifestyle Program Guidelines

Chapter 12   **185**

The Guerrilla Diet & Lifestyle Program – Introduction

Chapter 13   **189**

So, What Should We Eat… and Why?

Chapter 14   **239**

The Guerrilla Diet Shopping List

Chapter 15   **243**

Think and Grow Slim

Chapter 16   **247**

The 12 Week Guerrilla Diet & Lifestyle Program

Chapter 17   **263**

A 30 Day Example of The Guerrilla Diet and Lifestyle Program

Chapter 18   **279**

References

Introduction

When I was sixteen years old my parents got divorced, and my father, whom I was living with, had a new woman in his life. She cooked meals for my father, my sister and I, but her foods were different from the ones I had previously encountered. Her cooking involved much fat, and her dishes were rich with dairy products, especially cream and butter. Although this diet was very tasty for me, I was having difficulty coping with it and found myself increasingly gaining weight. This weight gain had a negative effect on my self-esteem and soon afterward I began a path of eating disorders that lasted a decade and a half and shifted my life around. Since that time, upon dealing with my first diet, I became interested in finding the ideal diet for human consumption. I researched and personally experienced practically every fad diet that came on the market throughout the years. I also looked into human eating habits, where they came from, and how these habits evolved. I was determined to change my life around and become more productive, healthy, and happy. But as long as I was suffering from my eating disorder "addiction," I was having zero success and my life was on a downward spiral.

At school I was an aspiring young athlete, specializing in the 800 meter run as well as running half marathons and marathons at a very young age. I had many issues about my body and did not have a clue as to what foods I should eat to supply me with sufficient energy for running while not gaining excess weight. I was eager to find the ideal diet for my health and my sanity.

At first I began researching psychological methods that would help me live a happy and fulfilled life and stop my addiction to

Introduction

food. The psychological methods I came across helped me conquer bulimia and later achieve my dream relationship and success in the financial field. I have put together these methods in my online course called "The Magic 8 Step Formula to Success, Happiness and Fulfillment – Your Secret Step By Step Guide To Get You Smiling and Passionate About Life Starting Today" which helped many people around the globe achieve these high ideals.

However, soon after another challenge entered my life in the form of cancer. In fact, I got it twice in two years. This is when I finally understood that the psychological methods and mind techniques I had mastered were simply not enough to achieve lasting success in the important field of health. These techniques were great for achieving financial and personal success in my life, but not good enough for achieving the lasting health I wished to reach. I felt that I needed to reevaluate my diet from my deepest core beliefs about nutrition, even though I was sure that my diet was good and healthy. After all, I held a Bachelor of Science (BSc) degree in Nutrition and Biochemistry, and a Master of Science degree (MSc) in Medical Science and many diplomas in alternative medicine. I felt I knew a fair amount about the body's nutritional needs, but apparently this was not the case. I finally understood that to achieve lasting health I would need to follow the laws of nature.

Now, at the start of my doctoral research program, after twenty-six years of substantial nutrition, immunology, and medical university studies, as well as extensive college studies in chemistry, biochemistry, alternative nutrition, and other alternative health practices, as well as reading countless books, publications, research articles, and studies throughout my adult life, and performing my own research study titled "The Lee Village Study," I can safely say that I have found the ideal diet and lifestyle program. It promotes lasting health and mental agility, rids us of unwanted diseases, both physical and mental, and gives us a feeling of vibrant energy as well as control over our health and happiness.

I am overjoyed to present before you the healthiest diet and lifestyle program for humans: ***The Guerrilla Diet and Lifestyle Program.***

Introduction

In fact, this diet is not really a diet, but rather a total lifestyle program that is backed by much solid evidence from many different scientific fields combined, including genetics, evolutionary science, zoology, medicine, and nutritional sciences.

This book holds the knowledge and step by step guidelines you will need in order to apply the ideal diet for human consumption along with precise lifestyle plans to support your own personal health, vitality, and longevity.

This diet has helped me change the course of my own health completely around.

By applying this knowledge to my personal life I have gained complete control over my weight issues as well as conquering cancer. Since then, I have provided the information found in this book to countless individuals whom have applied this knowledge to overcome heart disease, cancer, renal disease, and diabetes, as well as to achieve their ideal weight.

This dietary and lifestyle program will not only support you on your path to your own personal health, but also that of your future generations through epigenetics. I will go into this exciting relatively new field of research later in this book to show you how small changes in dietary and lifestyle habits can help you change the health destiny of yourself and your offspring.

Moreover, this dietary and lifestyle program is also healthy and sustainable for our environment and for our planet at large. This is the diet we were evolutionarily meant to consume as human beings and which holds the key to the lifestyle we are anatomically and physiologically designed to live.

This dietary and lifestyle program supports the health of our cells and promotes longevity and a life of peak health and thriving energy that we each long for.

The information in this book, once utilized, will help you reach optimum health at any age, which is your natural state. Nothing less than this is natural for us.

Now in my mid-forties, I look and feel better than I have in the past two and a half decades of my life.

Introduction

My children have also benefitted from being on this diet. My two eldest daughters have been mentally handicapped from birth as well as suffering from epilepsy. But following a total transformation in their dietary and lifestyle patterns, along with sixty other children with a similar medical background, this diet and lifestyle program is proving to be of great benefit not only for their waistline, but also for their cognitive levels and overall health. My two younger daughters are also learning the nutritional concepts that they need for life at a very young age which I hope will help them make the right choices to support their health, now and in the future.

By following the instructions in this book you will learn how to take full control over your health state and the wisdom contained herein will assist you in making the right choices to guide you easily towards reaching your ideal weight and optimal health.

Because this is the ideal diet for human food consumption, you will never feel deprived nor dissatisfied. It will take time, of course, to recall your natural state of eating. After all, the propaganda we're fed through advertising in all forms of media, fad diets, processed foods with artificial flavorings and coloring's and from copious suggestions by people around us that feel they know what is best for us but have no real proof will need to disappear from our belief system. It will take time to reprogram our mind, to shift from what we currently feel the urge to eat to what we should be consuming. Fortunately this book will teach us the methods that will help us overcome any difficulties, both physical and mental, that we may meet on the way towards achieving our optimal nutrition and health.

This diet will keep your interest levels high, especially once you start feeling the results it has on your health and your waistline. You will happily continue on the regimen and will readily consent to it becoming a part of your lifestyle.

The principles behind this diet will give you the tools you need to choose what foods are right for you in all situations. Once you have this knowledge, you will be steering your ship towards the port of your desired health and weight.

The world is governed by natural laws, and when we obey the natural laws of health, we will flow with life and bring to us the

Introduction

energy, vitality, and happiness that we were intended to have and deserve.

An Important Note Before Embarking on Your Journey

As much as I would love every person to read this entire book from cover to cover and to understand the principles behind every suggestion, I do realize that in the information age we are living in and being bombarded with too much data coming our way on a daily basis, it may be difficult for some of us to handle everything contained in this book. Some of us, as much as we would like to, simply cannot find the time to read and digest this much information. For this reason I have structured the book in such a way that if you just want to dig into the diet without reading all about evolutionary details of why this dietary program is best for us, then simply feel free to skip Section 1 of this book and go directly to Section 2 where you will find **The Guerrilla Diet and Lifestyle Program** outline.

You may also find some of the information more interesting or relevant for you such as chapters on physical activity, the importance of sleep, epigenetics, and neuroplasticity.

Feel free to jump to these chapters at any time. You do not need the background found in other chapters to enjoy the information found there, and later on if you do wish to delve deeper into the subject, you will be guided to exactly where you can find the information you seek throughout the book by going to the relevant references.

I wish you an enjoyable journey and believe that you will be in an entirely different place consciously regarding the foods you choose to consume after "ingesting" the knowledge found in this book.

The journey is long. Be prepared for a marathon. This is no sprint. In fact, the journey to better eating habits and an overall improved way of living is never ending.

Please join *The Guerrilla Diet and Lifestyle Program* community below to receive your special bonuses for buying this book!

https://goo.gl/v87JYI

You will also receive regular information and read the comments of likeminded people who want to improve their health in a sustainable and long lasting way. Can't wait to see you there!

SECTION 1

Evidence Based Background Behind The Guerrilla Diet and Lifestyle Program - The Best Diet for Human Consumption

Chapter 1

Why "Dieting" Doesn't Work

"What's wrong with extreme dieting and hard-core fitness plans is that they don't take into account the rest of your life."

— W. Alison Sweeney

"The meaning of insanity is doing the same things over and over and expecting different results." The quote above by Albert Einstein pretty much explains why the diet and weight loss industry are so wealthy.

People are looking in the wrong direction when searching for answers to solve their weight and health issues.

A dieter's mindset is the same mindset followed by most of the population: Once something is not in order, it's suddenly time to fix it. This mindset is one that focusses on taking care of the symptoms rather than addressing the cause of the problem.

Trying different dietary regimes is like sitting on a chair with thumbtacks on its surface. Every time you sit down you prick yourself and then have to bandage the wounds. Yet the following day you go back to sitting on the same chair again, ignoring the problem from the previous day until you once again experience pain and discomfort.

Chapter 1-Why "Dieting" Doesn't Work

This is what happens when we diet. We are focusing on the outcome instead of looking to change the causes behind the results we have before us.

Most people are not presented with very many other options, so they go with any new fad diet regime that they come across in the hope that this will be the one that will get them from where they currently are to where they desire to be. I know, because that's what I personally did for years. But every time we start on a new extreme diet which deprives our body of nutrients, we become stressed, which in itself has a negative effect on our health and prevents us from reaching our goal.

Research shows that more than 34.9% or 78.6 million adults and 17% of the youth in the United States are obese.[1] Furthermore, obesity-related conditions including heart disease, stroke, Type 2 diabetes, and certain types of cancer are all on the list of leading causes of death. Research proves that these are mostly preventable deaths. [2, 3]

The estimated annual medical cost of obesity in the US was $190 billion in 2012; the medical costs for people who are obese were $1,429 higher than those of normal weight. [4] In America, if the obesity rates continue to rise on their current path, the number of new cases of Type 2 diabetes, coronary heart disease and stroke, hypertension and arthritis could increase by ten times that number by 2020, and double again by 2030. [5] Obesity has risen by 34% since 1960, and morbid obesity (BMI above 40) has risen six fold to 6%. [4] According to the Boston Medical Centre, approximately 45 million Americans diet each year and spend $33 billion on weight loss products in their pursuit of a trimmer, fitter, healthier body. [6] But the products and diet information available mostly contradict one another. Some diets say that you should consume only fats to actually lose weight, while others say that fats are bad for you and you should go on a low-fat diet instead. Some diets look into food combining without any consideration as to what is being consumed, while others are so restrictive that they are completely boring and impossible to follow in the long term. Some diets say not to eat at night, while others say that only the total amount of calories

Chapter 1-Why "Dieting" Doesn't Work

consumed in a twenty-four hour period is what is important. This is very confusing to any person wanting to lose some weight, get fit, and become healthy.

Some people nowadays are even looking towards fad pills, powders, medications, or surgery to help them solve their weight and health problems. However, these options are still only caring for the result (the ill health and the weight problem), and ignoring the cause behind the result.

It is actually quite crazy that most of us forget to consider for a moment the reason behind our obesity or health state, and spend hours (and hard-earned dollars) searching to find quick and easier solutions to our problems. However, it is only by looking and examining the core reason for the problem that we can find a way to fix it.

The reasons why we have detoured off the path to wellness, longevity, and optimal health are due to two factors:

A. We have, through our choices, created an unhealthy environment for our cells to live and grow in.
B. We have allowed our core belief system about nutrition and health to be strongly influenced by the media which has its interest in monetary gain rather than our health at hand.

Only by going back to our natural state and following the natural laws of nature will we be able to take back what is lawfully ours and to start living the healthy life we deserve.

As I mentioned, I, personally, have been on every fad diet that I can think of from diets based on blood type, food combining, raw food diets, Atkins and so on. But at the end of the day, I never understood why certain foods led to weight loss while others made me fat. In fact, by following the strict regimes specified in each of those diets, my obsession about food only worsened. I was round the clock busy trying to manage my diet and weight. All of my spare time was wasted by conforming to my eating disorder and food addiction, so that I had really no time to enjoy life. Every waking hour was surrounded by thoughts of food. It was definitely a difficult and unproductive time in my life. The only industrious thing that I was doing at the time was improving food retailer's bank accounts! Only

Chapter 1-Why "Dieting" Doesn't Work

after becoming sick with cancer twice in two years did the idea enter my mind that perhaps my dietary choices were leading my health on a downward spiral! I never really found a sound concrete source of evidence based on a spectrum of sciences that shows the big picture as to which foods support human health and which do the exact opposite.

This is when I decided to use my excellent research abilities to learn what it is that humans should be eating to support our health and natural weight loss from a broad perspective. I learned that the most important factor for health and weight loss was the *choice* of fuel we use to supply energy to our bodies.

My research began by looking at the apes, gorillas in particular, due to our genetic and physiological similarities, in order to gain clues for the ideal human diet.

In the next chapter I shall cover what I discovered in my research of these fascinating primates.

Chapter 2

Why Human Needs are Different From Gorilla Needs Even Though Our Similarities

"There is no reason to teach an ape to become human. There are many reasons to teach some apes and some humans to transition the worlds between the species' boundaries, especially when our genetics are so similar as to make us 'siblings.' It is the way to learn how we become that which we are."

— Sue Savage-Rumbaugh

At the young age of twenty, I decided to examine the diet and lifestyle of gorillas and see what they ate and how they lived because gorillas are so similar to humans. They are one of our closest animal relatives (with the exception of the chimpanzee who are our closest animal relatives sharing 99% of our genes), although scientists found that in 30% of the gorilla genome is closer to humans than chimpanzees. [7] This is especially true in genes with accelerated rates of evolution for functions associated with sensory perception, particularly in relation to hearing and brain development. [8] I therefore decided to examine the gorilla's lifestyle habits to see what I could learn from them.

Chapter 2 - Why Human Needs are Different From Gorilla Needs Even Though Our Similarities

By examining the way these apes live and eat, and by taking a close look at their health and causes of death, we can conclude many things about modern human health and lifestyle.

Figure 1. Comparison Between Modern Humans and Gorillas

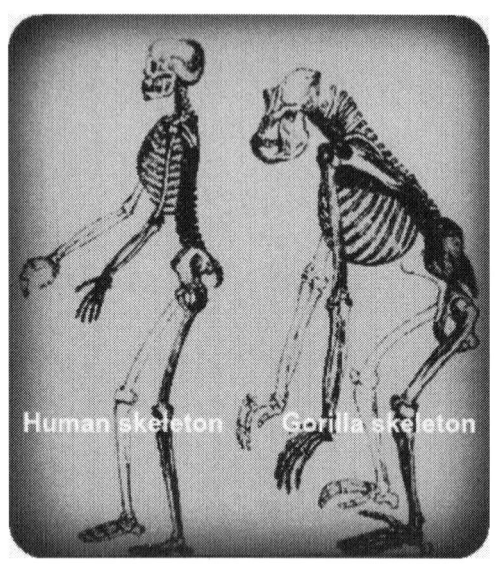

Gorillas share 98.4% of our genome and 99.6% of our DNA. The difference between gorilla and human gene sequences amount to only 1.6% on average, although there are further differences in how many copies each gene has. [9] This similarity in DNA may seem very surprising at first due to the obvious differences between man and ape, but nevertheless they are true. The difference we see between the species is due mainly to epigenetics. [10] Epigenetics is a relatively new field of science that examines how and why certain genes are expressed while others are not. (See Chapter 8 for a detailed look into

Chapter 2 - Why Human Needs are Different From Gorilla Needs Even Though Our Similarities

the science of epigenetics and how we can influence our genes using this science to make us slimmer and healthier.)

Humans and gorillas diverged from a common ancestor (Homininae) about 8 million years ago, [11] see picture on the following page.

Figure 2. This is our family tree.

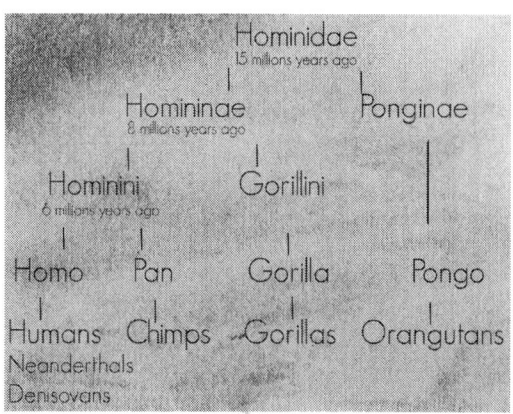

Gorillas are different from other monkeys for a variety of reasons: they are larger, they can walk upright for a longer period of time, they don't have tails and they have much larger, more developed brains.

There are three subspecies of gorillas today:
- Western lowland gorillas (Gorillas gorilla gorilla).
- Eastern lowland gorillas (Gorilla gorilla graueri).
- Mountain gorillas (Gorilla gorilla beringei).

The differences between the three gorilla subspecies are very minor and primarily consist of small variations in size and coloring.

Gorillas, like human beings, are intelligent, playful, emotional, and family oriented. They are even capable of learning

Chapter 2 - Why Human Needs are Different From Gorilla Needs Even Though Our Similarities

sign language. Sadly, despite our close relationship to gorillas, human beings have been the mountain gorilla's only real predators.

Let's look at differences and similarities between humans and gorillas:

Table 1: A Comparrison Between Modern Humans and Gorillas		
Characteristic	**Modern Adult Humans**	**Adult Gorillas**
Height	5'2" to 6 ft. (1.6 to 1.8 m)	Standing height, 4' to 6 ft. (1.2 to 1.8 m)
Average Weight	110 to 330 lbs. (50 to150 kg)	150 to 400 lbs. (68 to 181 kg)
Typical Close Family Structure	6 close members	6 - 30 close members
Gestation Period	9 months	9 months
Activity Levels	30 minutes - 2 hours a day	4-6 hours a day
Dietary Features	Omnivores	98% vegan
Teeth	32 teeth, 4 canines	32 teeth, 4 canines
Intestinal Anatomy	Longer small intestine, smaller cecum and colon	Shorter small intestine, larger cecum and colon
Brain Capacity	1200cm^3	350-400cm^3
Average Life Expectancy	70 years	35 years in the wild
Major Reasons For Death	Obesity, heart disease, diabetes, cancer	Human behavior and infections to a lesser extent

Chapter 2 - Why Human Needs are Different From Gorilla Needs Even Though Our Similarities

A Closer Look at the Facts:

Gorilla Vs. Human Physical Characteristics

Gorillas: Male gorillas are about twice as heavy as female gorillas in the wild and weigh 135–220 kg. (300–485 pounds). Male gorillas attain a height of about 1.7 meters (5.5 feet). A wild adult female gorilla typically weighs about 70–90 kg. (155-200 pounds) and is about 1.5 meters tall (4.92 feet). Gorillas, like humans, lack hair on the face, hands, and feet.

Humans: Today, males weigh on average 78 kg. (172 pounds) and attain an average height of 1.77 meters (5.8 feet). Human females weigh on average 67.9 kg. (149.3 pounds) and attain an average height of 1.63 meters (5.35 feet). [12]

In the past fifty years both men and women gained on average more than twenty-four pounds (11 kg.), while mean height increased approximately 1 inch (2.5 cm). Changes in mean body mass index (BMI) have also occurred. Between the early 1960s and the early 2000s, mean BMI for adults, both males and females between twenty to seventy-four years of age, increased from a BMI of just over twenty-five to almost twenty-eight. [12]

Gorilla Vs. Human Typical Family Structure

Gorillas: Gorillas live in stable family groups numbering from six to thirty members, most often eight members. The groups are organized and led by one or two silver-backed males who are related to each other, usually a father and one or more of his sons. Occasionally brothers lead a group.

Chapter 2 - Why Human Needs are Different From Gorilla Needs Even Though Our Similarities

The other members of the group include females, infants, juveniles, and young adult males. Adult females join from outside the group, and the young are offspring of silverbacks. The males dominate the group.

Humans: According to the Center for Disease Control (CDC), human family groups generally involve between four to ten people, including two partners, their parents, siblings, and children with whom close contact is maintained. (13)

In modern human societies, gender roles are not fixed, but constantly negotiated between individuals.

Gorilla Vs. Human Reproduction

Gorillas: Wild female gorillas give birth about once every four years starting at the age of thirteen. There is no fixed breeding season. Copulation may occur all year long in both gorillas and humans. The gestation period is about nine months, and births are usually single, though twins occur on rare occasions. A newborn gorilla weighs only about 4.5 pounds, (2 kg), and is utterly helpless for the first three months of life during which it is carried in its mother's arms. The young gorilla sleeps in the mother's nest at night and rides on her back during the day. Gorilla infants remain at the mother's side an average of 4.5 years. At this time the infant should already be weaned. Gorilla infant needs are identical to that of a human infant for the first year and half year of life. (14)

Humans: Most women give birth between the ages of twenty to twenty-nine. The average baby weighs 7.5 pounds (3.4 kg) at birth, however, a weight between 5 lbs. 8 oz. (2.5 kg) and 8 lbs. 13 oz. (4 kg) is also considered to be normal. (15)

Gorilla Vs. Human Brain Capacity

Gorilla brain size is 350-400 cm^3 in volume on average, while human brain size is 1200 cm^3 in volume on average.

Chapter 2 - Why Human Needs are Different From Gorilla Needs Even Though Our Similarities

Figure 3. Gorilla vs. Human Brain Capacity

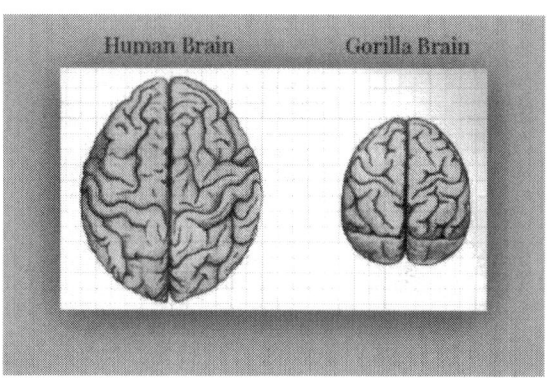

But are gorilla brains considered small in size when you look at primates in general?

No. The brain of a newborn human accounts for 10% of its total body weight. In adults this figure goes down to 2%. Gorillas have a much smaller brain to body ratio, but gorilla brains conform to the same neuronal scaling rules found in other primates, with a high density of neurons per volume and no increase in neuron size with body size. Research shows that like the human brain, the brain of the gorilla is built according to the same linear cellular scaling rules that apply to other primates. [16] However, it is the absolute numbers of brain neurons, regardless of brain size, that is a better predictor of cognitive ability than relative or absolute brain size. [17]

In the number of neurons, there is a major difference between gorillas and humans. Humans have roughly three times as many neurons (around 86 billion) than our close primate cousins (33 billion). Humans use 20% of the basal metabolic energy to feed the brain compared with 9% in gorillas. [18] Although large animals require less energy per unit of body weight, they have overall larger

Chapter 2 - Why Human Needs are Different From Gorilla Needs Even Though Our Similarities

total metabolic requirements to sustain their body. [19, 20, 21] The gorilla's larger body size offers clear advantages in protection from predators, and more success in competition with other species for food and territory. Large gorillas need to consume more energy in the form of calories to satisfy the needs of their larger bodies, and they tend to eat more nutrient dense, but lower calorie plant foods, while humans need more energy in the form of calories to feed our large brains.

Gorilla Vs. Human Activity Levels

Gorillas: The gorilla is active during the day searching and collecting food by walking about on all four limbs with part of their weight supported on the knuckles of their hands. However, occasionally gorillas can and do stand erect. [22] They spend much of their time foraging and nesting in leaves. At dawn the gorillas begin their search for food with the adults settling down to rest and nap in the late morning while the youngsters play.

The group travels a few hundred meters between several daily feeding bouts amounting to much physical activity throughout the day. Each group wanders through their home range of 2–40 square kilometers (three-quarters to sixteen square miles), and several different groups may share the same part of the forest. [10]

At dusk, nest building begins, and each gorilla builds its own sleeping nest by bending branches and foliage. A new nest is built most nights. Gorillas go to sleep at sundown and require on average eight to nine hours of sleep.

Humans: In modern society, most people are considered sedentary during most of their waking hours. In this category you may include most office workers who get little or no exercise on any given day. Moderately active people, such as construction workers or people running a minimum of one hour a day, share the same activity level as most gorillas.

Chapter 2 - Why Human Needs are Different From Gorilla Needs Even Though Our Similarities

There are a few groups of people considered to be vigorously active, among them competitive athletes and again, some construction workers. However, due to the invention and takeover of machines in most fields of construction work, this group of people is becoming smaller and smaller. [15]

Humans also need an average of eight hours of sleep a night. Due to the hectic Western world lifestyle, the average night's sleep of many people is reduced to six hours and this has a major effect on human well-being.

Gorilla Vs. Human Dietary Features

Gorillas: The gorilla diet is vegetation for all subspecies of gorillas and includes leaves, stalks, shoots, seeds, stems, and fruit, as well as around 2% to 3% animal protein from termites, ants, and caterpillars.

An adult male gorilla may consume more than 18 kg. (40 lbs.) of vegetation per day. [24]

Gorillas do not overexploit an area for food. They cut the vegetation in a manner that allows for quick replenishment to occur.

Gorillas rarely drink in the wild because they consume succulent vegetation that is composed of 50% water, and in the mornings it is covered with dew. Gorillas also wade waist-deep into swampy clearings to feed on aquatic plants to supplement their diets with iodine.

Humans: Humans are omnivores, capable of consuming a wide variety of plant and animal substances. [25, 26] Human diets vary according to available food sources in the regions of habitation, and also according to cultural and religious norms. Human groups have adopted a wide range of diets, from purely vegan to primarily carnivorous.

Until the development of agriculture approximately 10,000 years ago [27] which substantially altered both the human diet and the human population at large, early humans employed a hunter-

Chapter 2 - Why Human Needs are Different From Gorilla Needs Even Though Our Similarities

gatherer method of food collection. This involved the collection of fruits, grains, leaves, stalks, shoots, seeds, stems, tubers, mushrooms, honey, and insect larvae, along with the consumption, at times, of wild game that was either hunted in order to be consumed, or found dead and scavenged.

It has been suggested that humans have used fire to prepare and cook food since the time of *Homo erectus* [28] around 1.5 million years ago. However, there is no clear-cut evidence for this statement from archaeological sites, and most researchers agree that humans did not control fire until around 400,000 years ago. Nevertheless, it is known that *Homo erectus* did consume meat occasionally. It is suggested that when meat was consumed, it was eaten raw, as practiced even by some modern humans, and thus cooking cannot be presumed. (You can read more on this subject in Chapters 3 and 6).

Dairy farming began around 7000 years ago which allowed for a selected population to genetically sustain their ability to digest lactose (the sugar found in milk) into adulthood. [29] (More on this subject can be found in Chapter 7.)

Gorilla Vs. Human Teeth

Adult humans have thirty-two teeth, just as gorillas do. Gorillas have large strong teeth adapted for the coarse vegetation they consume. They are herbivores meaning that they feed on plants. Some herbivores have lost their canine teeth and have an empty space in their place. Gorillas, however, have kept their canine teeth which show their importance even in consuming a vegetarian diet, and that canine teeth are not there for the sole purpose of tearing meat. Gorillas have four canine teeth as do humans. Adult gorilla males develop big, sharp canines as they mature.

Canine teeth are very useful for cracking nuts and for crunching stems, as well as being a powerful weapon used to scare enemies away.

Human's canine teeth differ from meat eaters canines in size and shape. Canines are often the largest teeth in the mouth, but in

Chapter 2 - Why Human Needs are Different From Gorilla Needs Even Though Our Similarities

humans they are much reduced in size in comparison with carnivores. This condition permits the side-to-side motion in the human chewing cycle. [30] Canine teeth of carnivore animals are not only longer, but also very pointed. [31]

Early man was found to have greater canine teeth than modern man has today, but as they gradually acquired the habit of using stones, clubs, or other weapons for fighting with their enemies or rivals, they used their teeth less and less to scare predators. Through natural selection, the jaws, together with the teeth, became reduced in size. [32, 33, 34] In 1939, Professor Gustav Heinrich Ralph von Koenigswald found the fossil of the upper jaw and roof of the mouth of *Homo erectus* in Java, an island in Indonesia, which not only had canines that projected beyond the level of the neighboring teeth, but also had a gap between the canine and the incisor teeth which presumably accommodated a large projecting lower canine tooth as well. [35]

Gorillas, just as humans, have two full sets of teeth during their lifetime. The first set (similar to human baby teeth) are lost and then replaced by a permanent set of teeth in adults.

Gorilla Vs. Human Intestinal Anatomy

Humans and gorillas have very similar digestive systems anatomically, in which the major difference is the size and processes that are endured within the digestive system. [36, 37]

The digestion system of a gorilla, (like humans), functions through four major processes in order to digest food for the highest nutritional value and maintain energy and health.

1. Ingestion of food (eating).

2. Digestion of food — the breakdown of food through mechanical processes using the teeth, and through chemical processes using enzymes and acid.

3. Absorption of food — which takes the nutrients from the digested food particles through the villi of the digestive

Chapter 2 - Why Human Needs are Different From Gorilla Needs Even Though Our Similarities

system walls and into the bloodstream to be dispersed to the organs where these nutrients are needed.

4. Excretion — the removal of wastes, toxins and unused material.

It is found that the digestive system of all species goes through a process of plasticity, allowing the anatomies of the gastrointestinal tract and digestive system structures to change as a result of adaptations to environmental pressures found within their habitat. Environmental pressures include chemical, physical, and nutritional properties of their diet. These evolutionary adaptations show a relationship between diet and the structure of the digestive tract.

Gorillas: Gorillas, being herbivores, need to break down the cellulose they consume from plants they eat and absorb from it as much nutrition as possible. For this purpose, gorillas have larger colons than humans do (three times the size), with large amounts of bacteria and enzymes which destroy harmful pathogenic microorganisms and help them to metabolize foods that are otherwise difficult to break down, such as cellulose, through anaerobic (in the absence of oxygen) fermentation, allowing them to get as much energy from the cellulose as possible. [38] This breakdown process through colon fermentation contributes greatly to the success rate of the gorilla species due to the fact that potentially 57.3% of metabolized energy comes from short-chained fatty acids derived from the colon fermentation of fiber. [36] Gorillas have a relatively large and wide cecum (pouch) located at the beginning of the large intestine, hosting a large number of bacteria which also aid in the enzymatic breakdown of cellulose.

Humans: Early human ancestors used to have a similar intestinal tract to that of gorillas. We see this by observing the rib cage of *Homo erectus*. The rib cage protruded more and was very similar to that of a gorilla than to that of a modern man. Modern

Chapter 2 - Why Human Needs are Different From Gorilla Needs Even Though Our Similarities

humans have a smaller colon and cecum in comparison to gorillas. The previously larger intestinal tract helped humans metabolize cellulose more efficiently when early humans lived with the apes in the rainforest and ate similar foods to the apes.

The modern human cecum, known today as the vermiform appendix, averages eleven centimeters in length, but can range anywhere from two to twenty centimeters. Darwin suggested that our human ancestors became less reliant on cellulose-rich plants for energy, as they changed their foliage rich diets to foods more easily assimilated. [39] As the cecum became less necessary in the digestion process due to reliance on different food sources than were previously available in the rainforests, mutations that were previously harmful (and would have hindered evolutionary progress), became more and more frequent throughout the population. After millions of years, the once-necessary cecum degraded to be the small appendix of today's modern man (a sixth of the size of the gorilla cecum). [40] However, there is evidence that efficient cellulose metabolism still occurs in the large intestines of modern man. Researchers have shown that humans living in the Western world today derive 10% of their daily energy needs through anaerobic bacterial breakdown of fiber in the large intestine. This proportion is increased in people living in the third world. [41]

Humans have a larger small intestine compared to gorillas (3.5 times the size) to compensate for the small cecum. The role of the small intestine in digestion is absorption of nutrients and minerals found in food.

The structural differences between apes and humans go to show that the gut is flexible, and variation in dietary patterns can lead to structural changes of the digestive system.

Gorilla Vs. Human Cognition

Gorillas: Cognitively, gorillas lack the curiosity and adaptability of humans, but captive gorillas have shown a capacity for problem solving and have demonstrated a degree of insight as well as

Chapter 2 - Why Human Needs are Different From Gorilla Needs Even Though Our Similarities

memory and anticipation of experiences. They appear to be very skillful at learning sign language from humans. Some gorillas can recognize their image in a mirror and thus are said to have some sense of self-awareness. This is a trait that almost no other non-human animal possesses. (42)

Humans: Anthropological studies explain that the evolutionary success of humans is derived from a relatively larger brain with more neurons and a particularly well-developed neocortex, prefrontal cortex, and temporal lobes which enable high levels of abstract reasoning, language, problem solving, sociality, and culture through social learning.

Humans are the only extant species known to build fires and cook their food. (43) Humans also use tools to a degree incomparable to any other animal and are the only extant species to dress themselves with clothes and create and use numerous other technologies and interest themselves in the arts.

Gorilla Vs. Human Behavior

Gorillas: Gorillas are generally calm and nonaggressive creatures unless they are disturbed. (44)

Humans: Human behavior depends to a great extent on how people perceive a situation and what they expect to gain from it. Humans can choose their attitude and thus their social behavior. (45)

Gorilla Vs. Human Life Expectancy

Gorillas: The life expectancy of wild gorillas is about thirty-five years. Gorilla childhood mortality rate is 50% and this statistically lowers the average life span. Captive gorillas generally live well over fifty years. The major factors that contribute to gorilla's endangered status are mostly due to the effects of human behavior. Humans are the gorilla's main predator committing gorilla

Chapter 2 - Why Human Needs are Different From Gorilla Needs Even Though Our Similarities

infanticide, poachers killing them for meat or trophies, and capture the young to sell as pets. Snares meant for small game wound gorillas, and lately, mountain gorillas have also become the victims of neighboring human warfare.

Human encroachment on their habitat leaves gorillas with no place to live, breed, or feed. Gorillas require a minimum foraging range to meet their dietary requirements. The more foraging range they have, the more dietary diversity they have.

Humans are destroying forests for lumber, farming, grazing, and expanding human settlements to meet the needs of the ever-growing human population, and this will only get worse during this century.

But aside from humans, the Ebola virus has also had a serious toll on gorilla population. [46] Their mortality rate from the Ebola virus is averaged to be about 38%.

Mountain gorillas also reproduce more slowly than humans.

Humans: During the Bronze Age about 5500 years ago (3300 – 1200 BC) and during the Iron Age (1200 BC – 500 BC) human life expectancy was only twenty-six years! [47] During the early 1600s, life expectancy slowly rose for those who survived life hazards (infant mortality accidents, epidemics, plagues, wars etc.) and ranged from sixty to seventy years, just as it was before the advent of agriculture when humans were hunter-gatherers, and before the ascend in human population. [48, 49, 50]

In the US, the average lifespan increased during the 20th century by more than thirty years, of which twenty-five years can be attributed to simple advances in public health, and the remaining 5% to advances in medical science. [51]

Gorilla Heath and Mortality in Captivity Vs. Human Health and Mortality

Gorillas: Western and Eastern lowland gorillas can survive in captivity: mountain gorillas do not. Currently there are less than

Chapter 2 - Why Human Needs are Different From Gorilla Needs Even Though Our Similarities

fifty gorillas residing within zoos. However, gorillas in captivity face other health problems.

When gorillas were first being kept in zoos in Europe and North America, they were fed the same kinds of food that the local people were eating instead of being supplied with foods that are similar to those found in their natural habitat. Gorillas were fed several servings of "nutritional cookies" a day made from simple processed "white" grains, sugar, and added vitamins with the good intention of ensuring that the gorillas received all of their nutritional requirements. Cookies were also given as treats to promote good behavior. In other words, gorillas were basically fed a typical Western world diet based of processed, calorie rich, and nutrient poor foods – a far cry from their natural diet in the wild.

As a result of their new life style, gorillas fell prey to the same kinds of illnesses that are the leading causes of death in the Western world in humans. These illnesses were rare among people from third world countries, especially Asia and Africa, and were unheard of in ape populations. Gorillas in captivity, fed the common Western world diet, showed a tendency in both sexes to grow obese, especially when fed diets rich in simple sugars and carbohydrates. Obesity was never observed in wild gorillas.

This change in diet and lifestyle led to the same effect they have on humans, and heart disease became the number one killer of gorillas in North American zoos. In 2005, after a twenty-one-year-old gorilla named Brooks died of heart failure at the Cleveland Metroparks Zoo, researchers started to take a closer look at gorilla heart health. [52] Captive gorillas were found to have high serum cholesterol levels, ranging from 281 to 311 mg/dl. [53] Researchers examined the possibility of the effect of diet on gorilla health. They noticed that gorillas were consuming diets that were very low on fiber and rich in meat and egg products, [54] a diet very different from the gorilla's natural diet. In the wild, gorillas consume foods that are very low on fat and protein, but very high on fiber. The gorilla's diet in the wild also changes seasonally. They consume less foliage and more fruit during the wet season. [55]

Chapter 2 - Why Human Needs are Different From Gorilla Needs Even Though Our Similarities

Zoo keepers also noticed strange behaviors among captive gorillas that were never observed in the wild, including regurgitating sugar rich foods and then re-ingesting them. This behavior indicates that the change in their dietary patterns leads to the formation of sugar addictions in captive gorillas.

From these findings, in 2008 the first steps were taken by zoos to begin to wean gorillas off the commercially processed biscuits, and replace the high-sugar, high-simple carbohydrate and high protein diet that zoos had fed gorillas for years, with a diet more in line with their natural diet in the wild. Vegetables and leafy greens became once again their staples, and the food was scattered about their enclosure so they were compelled to forage. This way gorilla's also became more active as they would be in the wild. This reduced the incidence of heart disease and obesity immediately and now gorillas in zoos are living longer than ever before, till around the average age of fifty-four years. [56]

The new diet was quickly copied by other zoos in Columbus, Toronto, and Seattle. [52] By switching the gorillas back to a diet resembling their own natural diet, they restored their health. It may seem like common sense that gorillas should be given their natural foods for consumption even while they are in captivity, just as it is also common sense that we humans should consume the natural foods that we were naturally intended to eat, even if we have the ability to manufacture other foods.

Humans: Changes in human environment have greatly affected mortality patterns, especially the decline in mortality from infectious diseases, which during the 1900s were considered the number one cause of death. Today mortality rates primarily arise from lifestyle choices and behaviors.

Nowadays obesity-related diseases are the major cause behind human mortality. Obesity, resulting from consumption of more calories than are expended, has led to many health complications and increased mortality. [57] Worldwide, over one billion people are obese, [57] and in the United States 35% of all

Chapter 2 - Why Human Needs are Different From Gorilla Needs Even Though Our Similarities

people are obese. In the United States an estimated 300,000 deaths per year are due to the obesity epidemic. [58] The spread of obesity has led to increasing incidences of cardiovascular disease, Type 2 diabetes, hypertension, certain cancers, and other morbidities. *While genetics can predispose an individual to gain excess weight, the environment must be conducive in order for a person to become obese.*

There has been an increase in the availability of food, especially high-fat, high-calorie processed foods, and not enough education about the effects bad food habits have on our health. There is also a recorded decrease in the amount of individual physical activity which has played an important role in obesity becoming an epidemic. [59]

According to the National Institutes of Health, obesity is the second leading cause of preventable death in the United States, close behind the use of tobacco. [60] Smoking remains the leading preventable cause of disease and death in the United States, [61] and is linked to diseases of nearly every organ in the body.

According to the American Cancer Society, [62] an estimated 589,430 people are expected to die from cancer in the United States in 2015. That's one death from cancer every fifty-two seconds! The World Health Organization (WHO) estimates that global cancer diagnoses will rise from 14 million to 22 million people per year over the next two decades. WHO cites tobacco, obesity, physical inactivity, and alcohol use as the main reasons for deaths from cancer.

Heart disease is responsible for one in every four deaths, about 600,000 deaths per year in the United States alone. [63] Heart disease is the leading cause of death for both men and women of which coronary artery disease is the most common type of heart disease. [63]

Just as with gorillas, there are dramatic differences between mortality rates of men and women. [63] There are various reasons behind this gender difference in mortality rate, including risk-taking behaviors and occupations and higher suicide rates. [64] Males also report higher use of alcohol and tobacco. [65]

Chapter 2 - Why Human Needs are Different From Gorilla Needs Even Though Our Similarities

To conclude, gorillas are dying in the wild due to encroachment of humans into their habitat, leaving them with less and less land to reproduce and feed, while humans are dying mainly due to our own unfavorable lifestyle choices and behaviors.

We can change both of these statistics.

Chapter 3

An Evolutionary Perspective on Human Diet and Lifestyle

"The greatest tragedy of life is that it must be lived forwards and can only be understood backwards."

— Kierkegaard

If we are to consider our current eating habits without examining human history from the beginnings of mankind, we are doing great injustice to the subject. It is like looking for a solution for a problem without using the vast information we have collected throughout our lifetime. We would certainly not find the best solution for our problems under such circumstances. This is what fueled my research into human evolution from the beginnings of mankind. I wanted to find real answers and not blindly accept the often biased information available. I wanted to combine information from all of the sciences to get the whole and true picture for our best health and dietary choices.

So let's take a look at human evolution. Human evolution is a process that occurred over millions of years leading up to the appearance of modern humans. Evolution is a process by which organisms change over time as a result of changes in heritable genes (DNA), or in physical or behavioral traits.

Chapter 3 - An Evolutionary Perspective on Human Diet and Lifestyle

So where did we come from? There are two popular answers to this. One is the scientific evolutionary theory preferred by scientists, and the other is the religious belief shared by religious people. I see that both theories can coexist quite well, however, that is a subject best left for another book. This book is based on scientific evidence, therefore I will examine the existing scientific evidence of our evolution and how we can use this knowledge to improve the quality of our lives as well as that of our planet, and the quality of life of our fellow creatures who share this planet with us.

A Very Short Timeline Summary of Human Evolution

375 million years ago the earth began to assume recognizable forms. The earth's climate was warm and more humid at this time and remained so for the next 360 million years. It is at this time that the link between land animals and fish was determined. Scientists show that all animals who are walking on four and two feet come from a specific fish known as Tiktaalik roseae. This fish is believed to have been the first to have made the transition from the sea to the land. Tiktaalik roseae had similar limb bones to land animals, although on a different scale and in a different shape.

It is believed that reptiles have evolved from this ancestor, who later branched off into two groups 256 million years ago; one group remained reptiles or became birds, and the other group became mammals.

The earth then suffered from a mass extinction event which eliminated over 90-95% of marine animals. Land animals were not as seriously affected, but life on land took 30 million years to completely recover. [66]

From the second group that branched off to become mammals, another group diverged 85 million years ago to become primates.

Then the earth suffered another major extinction event which eradicated about half of all animal species, including all of the dinosaur reptiles, but excluded their descendants, the birds. [67, 68] It is at this time that mammals become the dominant species on earth.

Finally, 15 million years ago, the great apes evolved from their ancestors, the lesser apes, to form the homininae lineage which eventually led to modern humans. [69, 70]

Around 10 million years ago, the Earth's climate entered a cooler and drier phase and stayed that way until about 15,000 years ago. This further led to the transition to bipedalism, the transition from walking on four legs to walking on two feet.

Early Humans Separate from the Apes Six Million Years Ago

Looking at our family tree in the picture in Chapter 2 we can see that the emergence of modern humans (*Homo sapiens)*, evolved from a distinct species of great apes of the homininae lineage 8 million years ago, which included 2 species of chimpanzees (*Pan*), 2 species of gorillas (*Gorilla*), 1 human species (*Homo*), and 2 species of orangutans (*Pongo*). [71] Molecular evidence suggests that apes split off from the lineage that eventually led to modern humans sometime between 8 and 6 million years ago.

The earliest fossils that have been argued to belong to the human lineage, hominins, after the split from the apes belong to an extinct species *Sahelanthropus tchadensis*, which dates back to 6 million years ago. [72, 73] The fossil skull shows that its brain size was only 320 cm^3 to 380 cm^3 in volume, similar to the brain size of gorillas, and much smaller than an average modern human brain of 1200 cm^3. [74]

Early Humans Become Bipedal (Walk on Two Limbs) Five Million Years Ago

While still living in the rain forests with the other apes, hominins became bipedal (walking on two limbs), which offered them an advantage in long-distance travel between tree clusters in the rain forests compared to walking on four limbs. [75, 76] This increased travel efficiency is likely to have helped in finding more food resources in the rain forests.

About 4 million years ago we see the next ancestor in the hominin lineage known as *Australopithecus*. *Australopithecus* evolved in eastern Africa before becoming extinct two million years ago. They were fundamentally bipedal and thus excellent long distance walkers. Their brains were roughly 35% of the size of that of a modern human brain. *Australopithecus* mainly ate vegetables and roots, as well as nuts and seeds. [77, 78] The most famous *Australopithecus* fossils found belonged to "Lucy," a 40% complete skeleton of a female discovered in Hadar, Ethiopia in 1974.

Global Weather Changes Force Early Humans Out of the Rain Forests To The Savanna Grasslands Two Million Years Ago

Major change within the hominin species began to occur 2 million years ago and it was a change in weather conditions that led to the appearance of modern humans on earth!

2.7 million years ago the earth's climate changed and entered the Ice Age, a series of freezing glacial events separated by interglacial periods of warmer temperatures. Each period of glaciation in the Ice Age lasted about 10,000 to 50,000 years. The most recent glacial period chilled the Earth just over 10,000 years ago.

One general consequence of the Ice Age was that the North African tropical rain forest began to recede and was replaced first by open savanna grasslands, and more further away, by desert (the modern Sahara desert). This affected the environment of hominins and primates. As rain forests receded due to global cooling, the savanna grasslands expanded. It was at this point that hominins and apes parted. Due to the hominin's ability to walk on two limbs they had the necessary capabilities to leave the receding rain forests for life on the growing Savannah. Gorillas remained in the shrinking rain forests where they still live to this day. (79, 80)

Early Humans Are Forced to Change Their Dietary Patterns after Arriving On The Savanna

Upon leaving the rain forests for the savanna, hominins needed to change their dietary practices. Herbaceous leaves that were plentiful in the rain forests were sparse on the savanna, forcing hominins to start feeding on other foods.

Hominins adaptability to climate change and ability to exploit new kinds of habitats for food gave them the edge over other species. (81) It was these evolutionary changes which stimulated the evolution of bigger brains in early humans, making them eventually smarter and leading to the success of the species.

During the next few centuries we observe a steady process of brain growth. We see this in the next ancestor of the genus *Homo*, *Homo ergaster,* whose brain was on average 50% larger than his predecessor.

Homo ergaster were therefore smarter than their predecessors. *Homo ergaster* also began shedding their hair, making them bare skinned in comparison with the apes. This helped them to disperse excess heat through sweating giving them an edge in the hot Savannah. The larger brain and the more advanced skills allowed *Homo ergaster* to thrive in the hostile savanna environment previously too daunting for primates. *Homo ergaster* had *a* jaw and tooth size closely resembling that of modern humans, and their fossils show that their digestive tract grew smaller suggesting that whatever *Homo ergaster* began consuming 1.9 million years ago, is what our bodies are still designed to consume today.

Chapter 3 - An Evolutionary Perspective on Human Diet and Lifestyle

What Was the Magical Food That Allowed Humans to Succeed As a Species?

So what did *Homo ergaster* eat? It is obvious that hominin dietary patterns changed after leaving the forests because food diversity was different on the savanna than in the rain forests. Furthermore we see a change in dental and digestive structures. Hominin brains became larger upon leaving the rain forests, and a larger brain requires more energy to fuel it. It is a metabolically expensive tissue and therefore it would have required a regular, high-energy, dense food source to support its growth under natural selection.

But what was this food that allowed for such a major brain growth spurt?

Was Meat the Magical Food That Allowed Humans to Succeed As a Species?

Was meat the food source that allowed early humans to survive on the savanna and to grow their brains to double and later triple the size of a gorilla brain?

At first it was suggested that this regular and high quality food source that hominins consumed on the savanna was meat. Since bones are better preserved than vegetable matter, they give the impression that hunted animals must have been a primary food source. [82]

Previously scientists considered hunting big animals as the distinguishing factor between humans and apes. Apes do not hunt. However, based on all of the evidence we have today, it is obvious that this was not the case. It is assumed that hominins may have, to some extent, consumed meat from dead animals which they found sporadically by scavenging. But meat from dead animals was not readily available and meat found on the hot savanna was probably full with parasites which made eating it quite dangerous.

Moreover, to be dependent on meat as a regular food source on the savanna, hominins would have needed to hunt the big game

Chapter 3 - An Evolutionary Perspective on Human Diet and Lifestyle

that roamed the savanna themselves looking for fresh meat. To hunt big game successfully, hominins would have needed to master the skill of hunting, one that requires much planning. They would have also needed to create tools to throw stones that would travel long distances since animals would learn to keep a distance from their predators.

Throwing is a very complex activity that requires thought and planning. Animal prey moves and does not remain in one spot waiting to be hit, making this skill even more complex to attain. Gorillas hardly have the ability to throw anything. [83] Hominins needed to get better at throwing before hunting would be possible, since when you throw something at a target and miss it, the animal runs away and learns to be more careful the next time. Hunters must use a wealth of information to make context-specific decisions, both during the search phase of hunting and then after prey is encountered. These skills, which have a very long learning curve, were not developed in these early hominins. Evidence shows that this skill was mastered only 1 million years later, perhaps due to lack of language at that time. [84, 85] Furthermore, stone tools were very basic at the time and not advanced enough to kill large animals in one shot.

Anthropologists tend to agree that due to natural limitations hominins may have encountered in hunting, meat consumption was occurring too sporadically to have been the cause behind the increase in brain size and the survival of our species. Evidence also suggests that the large animals roaming the savanna were a very poor food source for hominins. Their meat was lean with almost no fat and the protein levels were too high to consume in abundance, rendering their meat an inefficient source of calories, especially when consumed in excess.

In fact, meat could not have been eaten as a major food source prehistorically because dietary proteins, when consumed in excessive amounts, become toxic to the body. Keep in mind that **the capacity of protein digestion is limited.** We can only metabolize somewhere between 200 and 300 grams of protein per day, and protein consumption exceeding this level produces toxic

Chapter 3 - An Evolutionary Perspective on Human Diet and Lifestyle

waste that our bodies have difficulty in eliminating. Furthermore, some of the protein consumed would be used for cellular growth and repair and wouldn't be available for energy, therefore protein is an inefficient energy source. [86] In fact, 250 g of protein provides only 1000 calories! That's not nearly enough to sustain even a modern day sedentary adult at room temperature, let alone an active hunter-gatherer living on the harsh African savanna! Furthermore, it is well documented that people who eat too much lean protein and not enough fat end up in a situation called "rabbit starvation" or "mal de caribou," [87] whereby ammonia builds up in the blood. If this continues, the person will suffer from diarrhea and mineral losses and will eventually die. There is much literature on African explorers who tried to survive on the African Savannah on meat protein, but the animals were so lean that the explorers became very sick from consuming high amounts of lean meat. [88, 89, 90]

Moreover, a person who consumes a diet rich in animal protein will experience higher metabolic costs than those whose diet is composed primarily of carbohydrates, or fat, or protein from vegetable sources. In fact, a sedentary adult surviving on hunted meat would require half their calories from fat, and an active hunter would require three-quarters or more of their calories from fat in order to survive.

Richard Wrangham, a British primatologist and anthropologist with a keen interest in Human Evolutionary Biology, calculated that hominins living on the savanna with bigger brains would need to consume approximately 12 pounds (5.5 kg) of raw plant food a day to get enough calories to survive, and if they were also eating raw meat, chewing it would require enormous amounts of energy. The hypothesis that the addition of high-energy raw meat to the hominins' diet is responsible for the increase in their brain size therefore cannot be true. Wrangham claims that hominins would have needed to chew raw meat for 5.7 to 6.2 hours a day, or raw meat and vegetables for 7 hours a day to fulfil their daily energy needs. Hominins at the time had low and flat teeth as we do today, which are not designed to eat raw meat quickly. [91]

Chapter 3 - An Evolutionary Perspective on Human Diet and Lifestyle

John D. Speth, a Professor of Anthropology in the Department of Anthropology and Curator of North American Archaeology in the Museum of Anthropology, looked at the role of big game hunting among modern hunter-gatherer groups (the San and Hadza) so as to understand ancient human hunting practices. Speth questioned the long-standing view that big game hunting evolved primarily as an effective and reliable food source for hominins after they left the African rain forests where they resided with the apes.

The Hadza people of Africa are a hunter-gatherer society that currently lives much like their ancestors lived for thousands or even tens of thousands of years. [92] They are the last full-time hunter-gatherers in Africa and they forage for food. Hadza men specialize in procuring meat, honey, and baobab fruit. Women specialize in gathering tubers, berries, and greens. [93] The Hadza adjust their diet according to season and circumstances.

During the wet season, their diet is composed mostly of honey, some fruit, tubers, plant foods, and very rarely meat. The contribution of meat to the diet increases during the dry season, although certainly not to the levels of daily consumption we are accustomed to in most Western cultures. During the dry season, the game is concentrated around water sources. [94] The Hadza men go out to hunt during the dry season, but even then they rarely bring home meat to offer their wives and children. It was observed that the Hadza men fail to catch meat 97% of the times they go out hunting. Furthermore, they share the meat mainly with their co-hunters at the site of the hunt and less with their family. Hunting actually increased during times when staple foods were in abundance during the dry season. The staple food in abundance during this time comes from the baobab tree which ripens only in the dry season. The women are the gatherers, and during the year they bring home over 80% of the food consumed by the whole family. The men collect honey when food is sparse. [95] Honey represents a substantial portion of the Hadza diet and there is a nutritional reliance on honey (as well as larvae and bee pollen) when food is scarce. [95]

Speth did not understand the behavior patterns of the hunter-gatherers regarding hunting. [96] They would kill animals, but would discard much of their meat, and they would hunt during seasons when food was plentiful. Furthermore, they did not meet with much success during their hunting expeditions. His research came to the conclusion that the main reasons for hunting were actually related to rituals and a show of masculinity, bravery, courage, strength, heroism and boldness among non-kin, rather than hunting to provide a dietary necessity. [97, 98]

By looking at these primitive tribes, one thing becomes certain: their human diet focused much less on meat as a food source than we may have been led to believe.

It was only in the 1980's that scientists found more evidence that gave clues as to what foods early hominins were consuming. In 1984, anthropologist Richard Leakey and Kamoya Kimeu found a nearly complete skeleton of a *Homo ergaster* child believed to be between 1.6 and 1.7 million years old. Some scientists believe that *Homo ergaster* diverged from *Homo habilis about* 1.8 million years ago.

The skeleton of the *Homo ergaster* child, later referred to as the Nariokotome Boy, [99] comprises 108 bones, making it the most complete early human skeleton discovered. He had a brain size of 880 cm^3 in volume, already double that of his ancestor *Sahelanthropus tchadensis,* and that of gorillas and chimpanzees. In the fossil remains of the Nariokotome Boy, found near Lake Turkana in Kenya, we see evidence that already at this stage the gut had shrunken to a modern human-sized gut due to the shape of his ribcage.

What Does Our Brain Size Have to Do With Gut Size?

The brain is an incredibly expensive organ in terms of energy consumption. It uses 20% of our Basal Metabolic Rate (BMR) which is the rate of energy expenditure at rest whilst being physically and

Chapter 3 - An Evolutionary Perspective on Human Diet and Lifestyle

psychologically undisturbed and in normal environmental conditions.

Hominin brains grew so large through natural selection over a period of millions of years. Since brain tissue requires twenty-two times the energy of skeletal muscle in order to function, to accommodate this increase in brain size they must have had a good, high quality readily available food source.

But what was this regular food source which was easily accessible by early humans 1.7 million years ago, that allowed the growth of their brains to such large proportions and allow their digestive organs to become smaller?

The Four Magical Foods That Allowed Humans to Succeed As a Species

One food source that supported hominins after their move to the grasslands and savanna, grew at exceptionally high rates due to the lowered temperatures in Africa at the time of the Ice Age. This food source grew readily all year round and was very hardy. This food is legumes (seeds that grow within pods) belonging to the pea family.

Legumes can grow in poor soils, are very drought tolerant, and require full sun, unavailable in forests, but readily available in the savanna.

Another regular and stable food source was grains including barley, millet, and rice, which grew in the open grasslands near legumes.

The third regular and stable food source was what are also known as plants with underground storage organs. Examples of these include cassava, potatoes, yams, beets, onions, carrots, etc.

And the fourth regular and stable food source was fruits. Examples include fig and Baobab tree fruit.

The underground storage organs were hidden underground and had no other competitors on the African Savannah. Underground storage organs support the plant from underground; they store energy so the plant can grow and complete its lifecycle.

This energy is stored in the form of starch or other digestible carbohydrate, a rich energy source.

These underground nutrient rich parts of the plant are usually avoided by herbivores as they are more difficult to reach. Plants with underground storage organs grow in plentitude on the hot Savannah as a result of the dry and unpredictable climate where plants changed to store energy underground.

Starchy vegetables and plants rich in energy in the form of carbohydrates as well as nutrients required a smaller gut than the one the hominins had at the time. Due to the discovery of legumes, grains and underground storage organs as a fuel source, humans were able to fuel their erect and smaller bodies using a relatively smaller gut, by using foods sources with increased dietary quality from this moment on in history. [100] *This had many implications on the destiny of our species.*

Moreover, grains and underground storage organs as a food source had the advantage of being much less fibrous than foliage. Reducing dietary fiber seems an obscure thing to do nowadays, but our ancestors ate so much plant matter that their bodies had to spend vast amounts of energy just grinding away at their food. The switch to starchy foods allowed early humans to thrive with shorter guts which also required less energy to maintain. The excess in energy became available for the brain tissue growth, allowing it to eventually grow in both size and in the number of neurons, an indicator of intelligence.

Why Did Apes Not Have Access to These Magical Foods That Allowed Humans to Succeed As a Species?

During the time the hominins left the forests and encountered these new food resources they also formed duplicates of the salivary amylase gene (AMY1). Salivary amylase breaks down large, insoluble starch molecules into more soluble and successively smaller starches and ultimately maltose. The salivary amylase enzyme improves the ability to digest starchy, carbohydrate rich foods and benefit from their starch in a more nutritious way.

Chapter 3 - An Evolutionary Perspective on Human Diet and Lifestyle

A research team led by anthropologist Nathaniel Dominy showed that humans, who are avid eaters of grains, have more copies of the salivary amylase gene than any other primates. Extra copies of this gene help us to breakdown starches in grains more easily and turn them into available energy sources. The research team also found that humans have anywhere between two to fifteen copies of the salivary amylase gene, and that people with more gene copies have more of the amylase enzyme in their saliva allowing them to easily break down starches found in grains. The research team then looked to other populations for a link between gene copies and diet. They found that chimpanzees, which feed mostly on fruit, have only two copies of this gene and very low enzyme levels. If any population eats more starch, its members will gain more copies of the salivary amylase gene. Individuals with more than six gene copies were more than twice as common in starch-eating groups compared to groups with low-starch diets. [101] The number of gene copies is in direct correlation with the levels of salivary amylase we have in the mouth. This duplication is thought to be an adaptation to a high starch diet, [102] which I believe can be found already in fossils dating back 2 million years ago. Duplicates of this enzyme allowed early humans to metabolize starches much more readily in the mouth than gorillas could, allowing for a smaller gut. When the gut became smaller, the energy it previously required was transferred to the brain, because hominin survival at the time depended on it. They needed to think and develop better ways to adapt and survive in the harsher environmental conditions they encountered in the savanna and during the Ice Age. It was the feeding on these legumes, grains, and underground storage organs that allowed the brain to grow to double and later triple its size. The food source was regularly available, plentiful, and of high quality, and humans did not have to compete with other species over them, especially the underground storage organs.

Digesting more starch from grains was a good thing for human evolution. This was especially useful during times when food sources were scarce. In humans, most nutrients cross into the bloodstream in the small intestine, and 10-15% of nutrients cross into

Chapter 3 - An Evolutionary Perspective on Human Diet and Lifestyle

the bloodstream from the large intestine. The salivary amylase enzyme allowed the blood vessels in our cheeks to absorb sugar due to the breaking down of starch already in the ingestion phase of the mouth. By using the salivary amylase enzyme, humans could digest smaller foods and get sufficient energy from them. Also, stringy plants like sugar cane became accessible foods because humans could extract nutrients by sucking on the plants without swallowing the actual fibers. [103]

This strong link between gene copy number and diet is noteworthy because it shows another quicker route for evolution. Instead of waiting for a beneficial mutation to pop up, evolution can favor duplication of existing genes with useful functions. Extra gene copies simply increase the gene's function in the body.

It is a fact that during the first period of increased brain size we do not see advanced tool making, and I believe that the reason behind this is _not_ that they were completely lacking in the intelligence needed to begin making tools, but that there *was less need* for these tools since these early humans fulfilled their dietary needs with grains, legumes, and underground storage organs. Just as a side note, this period of large brains using very basic tools went on for another 1 million years. [104]

In 1993, more than 1,000 researchers participated in a study to draw worldwide attention to traditional African cereals. In the study scientists examined the ancient crops of Africa to open people's eyes to the potential inherent in the grains that were the gifts of ancient generations, and to bring them into mass production today so as to help remove Africa from starvation, malnutrition, poverty, and environmental degradation.

This research study was also intended to save these grains from extinction and bring Africa a food-secure future.

This study titled "The Lost Crops of Africa" was a product of the Board on Science and Technology for International Development (BOSTID). In it scientists examined the crops of Africa south of the Sahara, [105] the place where early humans came from. They wrote: *"Africa's Savannahs are probably the oldest grasslands on earth and have changed little during the last 14 million years. Humans*

Chapter 3 - An Evolutionary Perspective on Human Diet and Lifestyle

have lived there longer than anywhere else." The report comes to the same clear conclusion as I have; "Grass seeds have sustained humans throughout time." (105)

BOSTID's study director says: "Africa has more native cereals than any other continent. It has its own species of rice, as well as finger millet, fonio, pearl millet, sorghum, tef, guinea millet, and several dozen wild cereals whose grains are eaten from time to time. This is a food heritage that has fed people for generation after generation **stretching back to the origins of mankind**. It is also a local legacy of genetic wealth upon which a sound food future might be built. But strangely, it has largely been bypassed in modern times." (106)

But how were grains eaten if only 1.5 million years later fire was controlled and the first evidence of cooking appears?

It is true that some grains and legumes have enzyme inhibitors and cannot be consumed completely raw. Enzyme inhibitors stop enzyme reactions, and some legumes contain trypsin inhibitors. Trypsin is an enzyme involved in the breakdown of many proteins as part of the digestion process in humans and other animals. As a result, protease inhibitors that interfere with trypsin activity can have an anti-nutritional effect. (107)

Once grains and legumes that have enzyme inhibitors are soaked, even for fifteen minutes, their enzyme inhibitors are no longer functional. In fact, soaked seeds contain their own enzymes and so they actually require less energy from the body in order to be digested.

However, grass grains when they are young, are still soft and do not have these enzyme inhibitors. It is when they dry that these enzyme inhibitors may become more prominent.

Legumes, grain grasses, and underground storage organs were the staple food that allowed early humans to survive the harsh weather conditions, and supplied them with a regular, nutritious food. Dry legume seeds have also been discovered in a Swiss village that is believed to date back to the Stone Age. (108, 109)

Legumes, grains, and underground storage organs provide protein and complex carbohydrates as well as vitamins and minerals.

Chapter 3 - An Evolutionary Perspective on Human Diet and Lifestyle

Legumes provide iron, magnesium, phosphorus, zinc, and other minerals, which play a variety of roles in maintaining good health. [110]

Legumes are 20-25% protein by weight, which is double the protein content of wheat and three times that of rice [111]. While legumes are generally high in protein, and the digestibility of that protein is also high, they are often relatively poor in methionine, an essential amino acid. Legumes are therefore complemented by grains which are high in methionine, but low in the amino acid lysine (which is found in abundance in legumes). In nature they often grow adjacent to each other and form a complete protein when consumed close together.

Human Evolution Continues: 1.9 Million – 400,000 Years Ago

The hominin lineage continued to evolve and *Homo erectus* diverged from the lineage of *Homo ergaster* immediately afterwards. The two species lived side by side until *Homo ergaster* disappeared from the fossil record around 1.4 million years ago.

Fossil skeleton and other fossil evidence suggest that *Homo ergaster* and *Homo erectus* had some kind of speech that would be recognized as a human voice. [112, 113]
They had the physique of the modern day human body, could easily walk very long distances, and were socially more similar to modern humans than to any earlier species. [114] Physically they resembled the modern human body and may have been the first ancestors to make and wear clothing of some kind.

Homo erectus along with Homo ergaster began spreading throughout Africa, 1.8 to 1.3 million years ago.

Homo erectus and Homo ergaster were the first hominins to live in a nomadic hunter-gatherer society, [116] in which most (or all) food was obtained from foraging wild plants and hunting few animals. *The Cambridge Encyclopaedia of Hunter-Gatherers* says: "Hunting and gathering was humanity's first and most successful adaptation, occupying at least 90% of human history until 12,000 years ago"... when agriculture began. [117] During their life span, *Homo erectus* learned to use his hands to throw sticks and stones which they used as weapons to kill small animals or as tools to crack open nuts.

Scientists suggest that early *Homo erectus* obtained meat via scavenging (feeding on dead animal meat found in their habitat), rather than hunting. [118] The meat they ate had either been killed by other predators or died of natural causes. [119] However, the bulk of their diet consisted of grasses, underground plant stems, roots, nuts, legumes, grains, herbaceous vegetation and fruits. [120] Their diets were made of over 80% plant foods, and they walked extensively over the savanna to gather their daily ration of food. It is assumed that they walked four to six kilometers (about two to four miles) a day to collect their daily energy requirements. [121]

500,000 years ago *Homo heidelbergensis* diverged from *Homo erectus* in Africa. They were intermediates between *Homo erectus* and *Homo sapiens* in Africa. The brain size of *Homo heidelbergensis* at the end of their period was 1200 cm^3 in volume.

The First Control of Fire

There is evidence that fire was first controlled by hominins about 400,000 years ago and this had a major impact on all parts of hominin life. This occurred at the same time that the Ice Age reached regular 100,000 year cycles of cold "glacial" periods and intermittent shorter warm "interglacial" periods. At this time we also observe another major growth spurt in cranial capacity in hominin fossils (from 800 cm^3 in volume to 1100 cm^3 in volume). [122, 123, 124, 125]

Fire allowed easier maintenance of body heat during the cold nights and opened the world to these ancient humans.

A recent discovery at the Wonderwerks cave in South Africa points to evidence that controlled fire may have begun much earlier, but most scientists agree that this fire was not yet used for cooking.

The First Migration Out of Africa

Chapter 3 - An Evolutionary Perspective on Human Diet and Lifestyle

A group of *Homo heidelbergensis* migrated to Europe and Asia 500,000 years ago when weather conditions allowed them to transverse the Sahara desert which became cooler during this time.

As *Homo heidelbergensis* migrated north and further away from the equator, they encountered harsher climate conditions and different food resources. "They had to be a little bit cleverer to figure things out," said David Geary, a professor from the University of Missouri. They had to find ways to feed, sleep, and keep themselves warm in different wetter and colder climates, as well as to protect themselves from different predators. All of this required planning and mental use of the mind to survive in this climate. This forced the brain to grow over centuries, just as today we see cortical expansion when one learns new motor skills. Today, the cortical expansion is followed by a period of cortical reorganization to make the most efficient use of brain size. During an evolutionary period of thousands of years of learning new skills we would see an expansion of the size of the brain. In fact, their brain grew to be over 250 cm^3 larger than the brain size of average modern humans today.

Professor Alan Walker, a paleoanthropologist who works on primate and human evolution, says in his book *The Wisdom of Bones*: "The speed of the territorial expansion of the *Homo species* is impressive, especially since geography, climate, fauna and flora would be changing all along the way... in fact, prey animals rarely expand their territories so far or so fast without evolving into a new species." [126] This is when we see the emergence of Neanderthals and Denisovans. The Neanderthals emerged from *Homo heidelbergensis* who migrated to Europe, and Denisovans emerged from *Homo heidelbergensis* who migrated to Asia. Both of these groups appeared around 400,000 years ago in the fossil record and their fossils have been found in Europe, the Middle East, and Asia.

Neanderthals were very closely related to modern humans, [127] differing only by 0.12% of their DNA. [128, 129] These similarities in genes strongly suggest that they interbred with human until they were absorbed into our species. [130]

Neanderthals were certainly not as primitive as we may have once believed. It is now known that they made advanced tools; [131]

Chapter 3 - An Evolutionary Perspective on Human Diet and Lifestyle

they were the first hominins to bury their dead; [132] they lived in complex social groups, and probably did have a language. *Homo heidelbergensis* moved into northern latitudes *without* the habitual use of fire and *without* the knowledge of how to cook their foods. It was only much later, in the Neanderthal age, about 300,000 years ago onward, that we find unequivocal evidence for regular human cooking. [133, 134] Hominin fossils from this time show proof of having smaller teeth and weaker jaws in comparison to their predecessors, and gorillas had much stronger jaws and larger teeth allowing them to feed solely on raw food.

The control of fire no doubt changed hominin eating and, sleeping habits, and habitation areas. [133] It is suggested that fire was used firstly to thaw food which was frozen most of the year, and later to cook food. [135, 136] It was previously believed that Neanderthals were primarily carnivorous; however, recent archaeological findings indicate that they consumed a raw, and later in history, a cooked mainly plant-based diet. [137, 138] Since it is more difficult to look for evidence of plant foods, there has been much less evidence on the plant component of early hominin diets until recently through the use of new scientific techniques.

In 2010, an isotope analysis of Neanderthal teeth found traces of cooked vegetable matter, [137, 139] and more recently a 2014 study of fossilized Neanderthal feces found substantial amounts of plant matter. [138, 141] The meat part of their diet, although limited, came from hunting and not from scavenging. It is suggested that they hunted very large animals in groups of males and females together, and would eat the fresh raw meat once they killed the animal. Professor John D. Speth, in his book titled *The Paleoanthropology and Archaeology of Big-Game Hunting: Protein, Fat, or Politics?* suggests that the reason behind their hunting may not have been for the sole purpose of meat consumption, but rather as a group ritual proving courage. Speth's research answered his longstanding question: "If large intakes of protein can be costly and risky to acquire, and above a certain threshold even deleterious to health, then why do hunters devote so much time and effort to killing big

Chapter 3 - An Evolutionary Perspective on Human Diet and Lifestyle

animals that yield protein in quantities that they and their families can't possibly consume safely?" [88]

Neanderthals had a larger brain size than hominins residing in Africa. It is known that Neanderthals were in an almost constant stage of starvation. This may have been what allowed their brains to grow to such sizes, because low calorie diets, cooking of food, physical activity, and learning new skills have been proven to substantially increase brain growth factors which support brain growth. [124]

Artifacts suggest that Neanderthals were sailing the Mediterranean Sea as early as 110,000 years ago. [142, 143] Neanderthals were also fishing in the Mediterranean earlier than their human relatives who were still residing in Africa.

Neanderthals became extinct or were absorbed into our species through interbreeding about 33,000 years ago due to their rhesus negative gene which gave humans the fore over Neanderthals during interbreeding. [144]

The First Appearance of Modern Humans 200,000 Years Ago in Africa

At around 195,000 (±100,000) years ago, the first evidence of *Homo sapiens* (modern humans) appeared. Early *Homo sapiens* took the place of local populations of *Homo erectus and Homo heidelbergensis* in Africa. The oldest fossil remains of anatomically modern humans are the Omo remains, discovered by a scientific team directed by Richard Leakey between 1967 and 1974 in Omo National Park in south-western Ethiopia. [145] The fossils show that they had the same anatomical build as we currently have today. However, they were still not as developed cognitively as the modern day human. [146]

Chapter 3 - An Evolutionary Perspective on Human Diet and Lifestyle

All Modern Humans Alive Today Come From Common Relatives in Africa

We evolved from early *Homo sapiens* some 60,000 – 160,000 years ago. [147] The hypothesis suggests that the female line ancestry of all present-day humans traces back to one single female, and the male line to one single male. To put this simply; all people alive today come from a woman who lived in Africa about 160,000 years ago, [148, 149, 150, 151] and from a man who lived 60,000 – 90,000 years ago in Africa. [152] This is proven through genetic material found in our mitochondria, the provider of genetic history in our cells which is inherited exclusively from the mother, [153] and the Y chromosome DNA which is paternally inherited. These two pieces of human genome are not shuffled through evolutionary mechanisms. Instead, these elements are passed down intact from generation to generation.

Speech and Modern Human Development 70,000 Years Ago

At around this time we find evidence for the origin of modern human speech in the region of south-western Africa. [154, 155]

The ability to speak and transfer information, which came about due to genetic mutations, had a major effect on the success of our species. [156, 157, 158, 159] These changes in our genome did not happen suddenly, but came about gradually with small evolutionary changes as a result of natural selection over a period of thousands of years.

But What Supported These Major Genetic Changes?

About 70,000 years ago a catastrophe occurred that may have led to the evolution of the human mind as we know it today, namely the super volcanic eruption at Toba, Indonesia. [160] It is one of the Earth's largest known eruptions. [161,162]

Early humans were unprepared for the sudden climatic change, and only the fittest and most intelligent of them survived and passed their genes onto the next generations. This led to a bottleneck of the human population around 70,000 years ago which led to a decline in the human population to less than 10,000 breeding pairs in equatorial Africa from which all modern day humans descended. [163, 164] This reduction in population allowing only the fittest and cleverest to survive set the stage for the advancement of our species. At this time the human brain reached its current size and form.

Modern humans have about 80 billion brain cells, but the size of our brains is not the only advantage that gave humans the edge over other species; it is the wiring of these brain cells that did. Humans have 100 trillion brain cell connections and this beneficial wiring is what supports intelligence.

Humans Migrate Out of Africa 60,000 Years Ago

60,000 years ago, came the earliest successful migration of humans out of Africa with living descendants. [165] This was made possible due to the earth entering a Mousterian Pluvial, which is an extended wet and rainy period in the climate history of North Africa. This period lasted 20,000 years and transformed what is now the Sahara desert into a grassland environment bearing lakes, swamps, and river systems. This allowed humans to cross the Sahara and begin dispersing all over the world to populate even the very northern continents. They travelled from Africa into Israel, and from there they spread to India, Sri-Lanka, and Bangladesh 60,000 years ago, and on to Australia 40,000 years ago. [166]

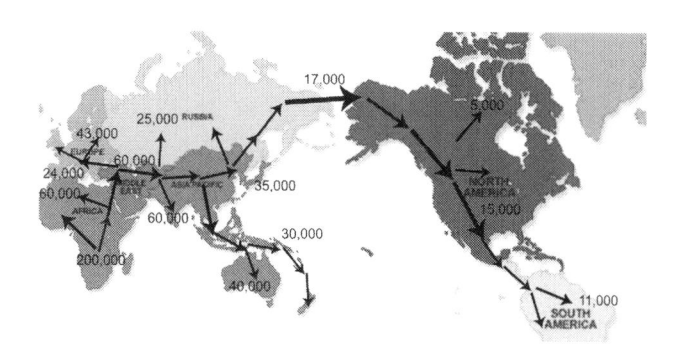

Figure 4. Humans Migrate Out of Africa

At 43,000 years ago we see the first evidence of modern humans in Europe. [167] When they first arrived in Europe and Asia, these continents were already populated by the Neanderthals and Denisovans who had arrived there with the previous migration out of Africa by *Homo heidelbergensis* about 400,000 years earlier. But eventually, as mentioned, over a period of ten thousand years, *Homo sapiens* completely displaced these populations [168,169] and remained the only living species of our lineage.

At 35,000 years ago we see first evidence of modern humans inhabiting Japan. [170]

At about 24,500 to 17,000 years ago humans inhabited Southeast Europe and Spain, Portugal, Andorra, and southern France. The Ukraine was then inhabited and shortly afterwards Russia. Around 15,000 years ago, the first humans reached North America, 13,000 km (8000 miles) away from their origin in Africa. They came to America by crossing the Bering Strait, a naturally formed, narrow waterway that connects the North Pacific Ocean and the Arctic Ocean, and lies between Alaska and Russia in Asia. (See arrow in Figure 5 on the next page.) Between 47,000 –12,000 years ago the Bering Strait became a land and ice bridge roughly 1,000 miles (1,600 km) wide connecting Asia with North America allowing

Chapter 3 - An Evolutionary Perspective on Human Diet and Lifestyle

humans to easily crossover into America. From 11,000 years ago it became a waterway again.

Figure 5. The Bering Strait between 47,000 –12,000 years ago

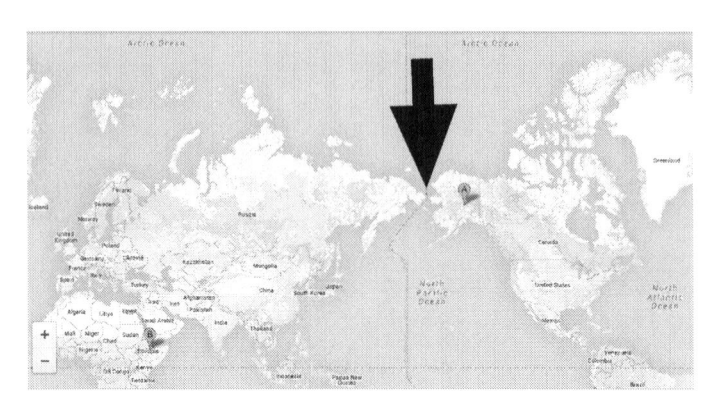

Figure 6: How the area around the Bering Strait looked 21,000 years ago

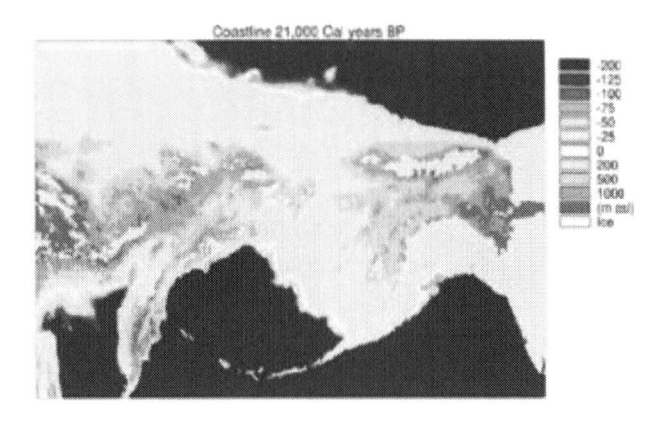

Chapter 3 - An Evolutionary Perspective on Human Diet and Lifestyle

Humans who entered the America continent travelled southward through Central America and reached South America 11,000 years ago.

At this time we see the earliest evidence of agriculture which completely changed human life on earth.

Agriculture and the domestication of animals marked the dawn of the Neolithic Era (the new Stone Age), around 11,000 years ago. The Neolithic era involved changes and a progression of behavioral and cultural characteristics, including the use of domesticated crops and domesticated animals. Unlike during the Paleolithic era, (the old Stone Age), when more than one human species existed (Hominins, Neanderthals, Denisovans, and Homo floresiensis living on the isle of Flores in Indonesia), only one human species (Homo sapiens) reached the Neolithic era. [171]

The Agricultural Age Begins Globally 12,000 Years Ago

We see the first evidence of agriculture 12,000 years ago in North East Africa and Israel. The first foods chosen to be grown through agriculture were grains, pointing to the importance of these foods in the human diet before agriculture, during the hunting-gathering period. Following shortly afterwards came the domestication of barley and peas, also very dominant foods during the hunter-gatherer era of our species. Next we have evidence of the cultivation of figs in the Jordan Valley, [172] as well as flax seeds, 11,300 years ago. [173]

Professor Jared Diamond, an American scientist whose research work involves a variety of fields including anthropology, ecology, geography, and evolutionary biology, explains that grains and legumes were easily domesticated from their wild ancestors because their wild predecessors required very little genetic change to convert them into a domesticated crop. Wild grains and legumes were in edible and productive form in the wild so they were easily grown by ancient farmers, merely by sowing or planting. Grains and

Chapter 3 - An Evolutionary Perspective on Human Diet and Lifestyle

legumes grew rapidly and could be harvested within a few months of sowing, a big advantage to people still on the borderline between being nomadic hunter-gatherers and settled villagers. They could be readily stored and were mostly self-pollinating. [174]

The domestication of crops is one of the first steps in moving towards a full-fledged agricultural economy. More plants became domesticated and their native characteristics were altered in a manner that they could not grow and reproduce without human intervention. A symbiotic relationship between the plants and humans developed, called co-evolution, because plants and human behavior's evolved to suit one another. In the simplest form of co-evolution, humans harvest a given plant selectively, based on preferred characteristics such as the largest, prettiest fruits, and reuse the seeds from the largest fruits to plant for next year.

Around 10,500 years ago, there was another very cold, abrupt climate change called the Younger Dryas. Here the glaciers covered Europe again, and some forested areas shrank while other completely disappeared. This period lasted for approximately 1,200 years, during which time people survived as best as they could.

After the cold lifted, about 9000 years ago, and the climate warmed up to temperatures that are similar to present day weather conditions, agriculture completely replaced the hunting-gathering lifestyle. Domesticating crops provided a reliable food source to feed the growing population. The nomadic hunting-gathering lifestyle could no longer feed such a large and growing human population.

In China 9000 years ago, humans began to farm rice and millet. [175] At this time there is also evidence of harvesting wild grasses in Asian Turkey and its surrounding area.

By 8000 BC, fully domesticated versions of einkorn wheat, barley, and chickpeas were grown, as well as the first evidence of domestication of animals. The first domesticated animals were dogs, descendants of wild wolves, which helped keep predators away, and as agriculture began they helped farmers control and guard the land. Sheep, goat, cattle, and pigs were soon to follow. They were first domesticated in the Zagros Mountains in Western Iran and spread outward from there over the next thousand years. [176] Domesticated animals were at first used for riding, transportation, pulling plows, and when they aged, for food.

The first stone-built structures were also built in the Zagros Mountains at this time.

Beans were first domesticated in eastern Mediterranean countries 7,000 years ago, and squash, beans, and peppers were domesticated in America 6,000 years ago. Soybeans, rice, wheat, barley, and millet were grown in China 4,000 years ago, and olives and fruits were cultivated in the eastern Mediterranean area 3,000 years ago. [177]

Agriculture Supported the Human Population Escalation

Crops were now farmed to meet the demands of the growing local populations which began rising dramatically.

Although grains and root crops were domesticated and cultivated in all the habitable continents, animals were only domesticated in a few areas on earth, principally in Western Asia where the earliest evidence was found for the domestication of sheep, goats, pigs, and cattle, followed later by donkeys, horses, and camels. Some forms of cattle and pigs, as well as chickens, were later domesticated also in south and east Asia, and cattle and pigs were domesticated independently in Europe. Very few animals were domesticated in America including turkeys and llamas, alpaca, and guinea pigs. Animals were not domesticated at all in tropical Africa or Australia! This is probably due to the abundant amount of grains, legumes and underground storage organs naturally found there which may have reduced the need to domesticate animals for food.

All of the farm animals and pets that are tame today, including dogs, cats, cattle, sheep, camels, geese, horses, and pigs, started out as wild animals, but were transformed over millennia into tamer animals.

In the next chapter we shall look at the effects of agriculture and the modern diet on human health, and compare it with the health of gorillas.

Chapter 4 - Dietary Requirements: Comparison Between Apes and Humans

Chapter 4

Dietary Requirements: Comparison Between Apes and Humans

"We are indeed much more than what we eat, but what we eat can nevertheless help us to be much more than what we are."

— Adelle Davis

      First we'll look at the content of a typical gorilla diet as this is where our roots lie. Then we will observe the evolutionary changes hominins went through discussed in the previous chapter. Lastly, we will look into the effects that leaving the nomadic hunter-gatherer lifestyle for agriculture caused whereby we began growing our own foods and domesticating animals for our consumption. We'll put these facts together to conclude the diet best suited for human consumption; one that is in tune with our modern day physiology, ensures an ongoing nurturing supply of energy to support our brains and our bodies, and maintains the health level we deserve.

Chapter 4 - Dietary Requirements: Comparison Between Apes and Humans

The Common Gorilla and Modern-Day Human Diets

The Diet of Eastern Lowland Gorillas consists largely of foliage, including leaves, stems, pith and shoots, while fruit makes 5-25% of their diets in contrast to mountain gorillas.

The Diet of Mountain Gorillas consists of over 142 different plant species. They consume foliage of herbs and vines, with leaves making up 68% of their food intake, stems 25%, piths 2.5%, epithelium from roots 1.4%, and the remaining 4% from bark, roots, flowers and fruit. During the rainy season, mountain gorillas eat bamboo shoots and mountain bamboos when they are green, young, and tender. The bamboo shoots are made of 84% water and therefore gorillas hardly ever need to drink water. During the dry season they eat many berries, especially blackberries that grow on high altitude.

Both Mountain and Eastern Gorillas have very flexible diets, [178] and it is thought that they consume a small amount of animal protein by eating small insects, insect eggs and larvae found on the plant foods they eat, although no evidence to consumption of animal matter was found in mountain gorilla feces. [179]

The Diet of Western Gorillas is the same foods as mountain gorillas, but in different proportions. Green plant material remains the majority of their diets; however, Western lowland gorillas eat more fruit [180]. About 67% of their diet is fruit, 17% is leaves, seeds and stems, and 2% is ants, termites, caterpillars, snails, and grubs. [181, 182] The Western lowland gorillas consume parts of at least ninety-seven plant species, and they also have access to aquatic herbs in some areas while they have less access to terrestrial herbs.

All Gorillas are very selective in their food choices, choosing only certain parts of the vegetation available to them at certain times of the year. [183, 184]

Gorillas prefer immature leaves over the mature ones, which usually contain less fiber, but more protein. [185, 186]

Chapter 4 - Dietary Requirements: Comparison Between Apes and Humans

The gorilla's diet in the wild is low in carbohydrates and fat, but very high in fiber which helps them to maintain normal cholesterol and blood sugar levels. When their diets are changed drastically in zoos and become rich in fats and simple carbohydrates, we see an almost immediate deterioration in their health state.

The gorilla's days are arranged around their feeding schedule. Gorillas normally have three rest intervals a day and they eat in between these resting periods. They spend a lot of their time traveling and foraging in search of food. Because plants and trees change with the seasons, they get plenty of dietary variation, plenty of rest, and also plenty of exercise during the day. Gorillas spend four to six hours daily being physically active. They only become dormant when it rains heavily.

The Diet of Humans living in the Western world on average consists of three main grains including maize, wheat, and rice, in their processed form stripped of their bran and germ layers. These nutrient poor grains form 40% of the diet. Meat, fish, eggs, and dairy products form 45% of the average modern Western world diet, and fruit and vegetables form the remaining 15%. This diet is a far cry from the one our bodies are meant to consume and to thrive on. Modern human diets are high in fat, low in fiber, and high in simple carbohydrates which is unsupportive of human health.

Gorilla and Human Energy Requirements

Full-Grown Adult Gorillas can eat up to 60 pounds (30 kg) of vegetation a day and walk about 4 km (2.5 miles) per day

Theoretically their energy needs can be fulfilled with 5500 to 8000 kcal/day. [187] To acquire this amount of energy, wild gorillas need to spend 50-90% of their waking hours foraging and consuming food.

When an animal or a human is hungry, their mind is focused only on finding food to satisfy their hunger. Thus gorillas in the wild that only consume vegetation are less likely to have the time when they are mentally free to develop other interests and skills. This is also not something they require for their survival while living in the wild. They need to protect themselves and have enough food to support their own nutritional needs and those of their offspring, as well as to secure their species for future generations.

The gorillas eat a very healthy diet that allows them to grow to a very heavy average weight of 150 to 400 lbs. (68 to 181 kg). Their large size is something that is important for their survival. The vegetation around them supplies all of the nutrients that they require for their health, including essential nutrients which are not produced within the body and thus must be obtained from their diet.

Adult Humans require on average 1900 kcal of energy per day. [188] This amount of food in the form of cooked food requires under 1.5 hours of chewing per day. This leaves us with almost 23 hours per day to be busy with other activities.

Gorilla and Human Essential Mineral Requirements

Gorilla essential macro-mineral requirements are similar to human essential macro-mineral requirements and include calcium, phosphorus, magnesium, potassium, sodium, chlorine, and sulphur which are abundant in their habitats.

The gorilla essential trace element requirements are also similar to those of humans, although little research on the qualitative or quantitative needs of gorillas for these elements has been conducted. In the wild, primates obtain minerals mostly from plant sources, although geophagia (dirt-eating) has been observed in mountain gorillas when iron was deficient in their diet. [189] This practice helps supplement the dietary mineral and trace element supply.

Green leaves are good sources of calcium and magnesium. Some gums are rich in calcium, magnesium, and potassium, and seeds and nuts are usually good sources of phosphorus.

The bioavailability of minerals in foods [190] for most species including humans is normally less than 100%. However, due to the fact that gorillas are colon fermenters, they have the ability to anaerobically breakdown foods with bacteria and enzymes, making nutrients more bioavailable to them.

Gorilla and Human Protein Requirements

Essential amino acids that make up proteins are required for the production of enzymes, hormones, transport proteins, lipoproteins, antibodies, and structural proteins which make up muscle tissue, connective tissue, hair, nails, and skin, as well as maintaining a normal acid-base balance and a proper fluid balance in and out of the cells.

Apes appear to have essential amino acids needs that are similar to those of humans.

It is necessary for both gorillas and humans to have a diet with sufficient protein to meet amino acid requirements.

If the body is deficient in essential amino acids from dietary sources, it is unable to build proteins and will have to break down muscle tissue in order to obtain the amino acids it requires.

Gorillas get their essential amino acids from vegetation rich in protein including bamboo shoots and young green leaves, woody lianas, bark (which contains up to 17% crude protein), epiphytes, and moss. These foods also supply them with a whole array of essential nutrients including by order of supply: Vitamins K, A, manganese, Vitamin C, fiber, calcium, choline, Vitamins B2, B6, iron, Vitamin E, copper, protein, magnesium, pantothenic acid, folate, omega-3 fatty acid precursors, Vitamins B3, B1, and potassium. Gorillas get enough vegetarian protein to thrive. They also obtain additional protein from the small amounts of insects they consume as part of their diet. Modern humans, as omnivores, can choose where we get our protein requirements. Whether from the vast array of plant based sources available or from meat products.

Chapter 4 - Dietary Requirements: Comparison Between Apes and Humans

Gorilla and Human Omega-3 and Omega-6 Fatty Acid Requirements

The wild mountain gorilla diet has a very low fat intake (3.1% of dry matter — the nutrients other than water found in food) in contrast with the diet of most modern humans. The Western gorillas have a fat intake of 14% from their total dietary energy intake due to the high fruit content of their diet. [191]

The overall fat intake from gorillas shows that saturated fatty acids account for 32.4% of the total fatty acids in their diet, while monounsaturated fatty acids account for 12.5% and polyunsaturated fatty acids (PUFA's) accounted for 54.6%. Saturated fatty acids have a more rigid structure because the fatty acid is "saturated" with hydrogen atoms and has no double bonds making it less flexible. Unsaturated fatty acids have at least one double bond making them more flexible than saturated fats. Monounsaturated fatty acids have one double bond; PUFA's have two or more double bonds.

Fatty acids are used by the body in the formation of cell membranes and storage lipids, like triglycerides. Fatty acids in membranes affect the structure and function of the membrane according to the type of fatty acid involved. The more saturated fatty acids in the diet, the more rigid and less flexible the cell membranes tend to be.

In the gorilla's diets, the essential PUFA's, linoleic acid (LA), also known as omega-6 fatty acids, and alpha-linolenic acid (ALA), also known as omega-3 fatty acids, were found in all of the seventeen staple foods they consumed regularly and were among the most predominant fatty acids in their diet: omega-6 – 30.3%, and omega-3 – 21.2%. Herbaceous leaves have higher concentrations of ALA, while fruit is higher in LA.

Dietary deficiencies in essential fatty acids and their long chain derivatives are linked to neurological abnormalities in humans and other mammals. [192, 193, 194] It is important to note that long chain omega-3 and omega-6 derivatives (including AA, EPA, DPA, and DHA) **are not essential** fatty acids because primates can derive them endogenously from shorter chain omega-3 and omega-6 fatty acids including LA and ALA fatty acids. In fact, consuming too much of the long chain omega-3 and omega-6 derivatives AA, EPA, DPA, and DHA, which come mainly from fish and meat sources, creates a risk for developing many modern day diseases. The reason behind this is that PUFA's are chemically unstable molecules and are therefore at risk of being altered and denatured by proteins and sugars. The combination of PUFA's with proteins and sugars create toxic by-products which can cause cellular damage. Since PUFA's are unstable fats, when they are consumed in large quantities and become an increasing portion of cell membranes, the cells themselves become more fragile and prone to oxidation. PUFA's in excess also contribute to the oxidation of low-density lipoproteins (LDL) to create a form of cholesterol transporter in the blood that's very unstable and atherogenic (promotes the formation of fatty plaques in the arteries).

Long-chain PUFA's are essential for proper brain, retinal, neural, and immune function. [194,195] The conversion of shorter chain fatty acids, LA and ALA, to their longer chain derivatives, AA and EPA, occurs readily, [196, 197] while the conversion to DHA occurs at a rate of only 1% in humans, [196] and this is likely to be similar in most primates. Despite the finding that the total percentage of AA, EPA, DPA, and DHA from all staple diet foods was only 0.6% in mountain gorillas, the high levels of the essential fatty acids LA and ALA in the diet suggest that the longer chain PUFA's are not limiting factors, and the wild mountain gorilla diet is not deficient in long chain PUFA's. In fact, if long chain fatty acids were limiting factors in the diet, then all animals would need to consume fish in order to supply them with sufficient levels of these nutrients which is not the case. In fact, **there is no need to consume fish to get sufficient levels of omega 3 fatty acids if the diet has sufficient ALA found in fruit, seeds, vegetables, and in green leaves.** The body will convert them to long chain fatty acids at just the rate and amount required by the body for optimum health. Fish produce these fats only once they feed on underwater plants rich omega 3 fatty acids. Therefore, omega 3 fatty acids in fish oils are actually plant-based products that come from feeding on omega 3 rich sea plants.

Chapter 4 - Dietary Requirements: Comparison Between Apes and Humans

Gorilla and Human Vitamin B12 Requirements

Vitamin B12 is produced only by bacteria. No plant or animal is known to produce this vitamin. However, many animals are able to concentrate and store the vitamin B12 produced by bacteria. As such, animal foods end up being important sources of this vitamin. Plants do not concentrate vitamin B12, so plant foods cannot provide this vitamin into our diet. The small (2%) addition of animal protein in the form of ants and larvae in gorilla's diets allows them to consume sufficient levels of B12 to meet their requirements. Only a very minute amount of B12 is necessary to meet the requirement for this vitamin in humans and apes. Ancient humans received sufficient amounts of this vitamin from the ground where the found their foods and in water sources. B12 is involved in the process of energy production. A deficiency of one or more of the other B vitamins may exacerbate the symptoms related to vitamin B12 deficiency. This is highly unlikely in gorilla's natural habitat, but common on a diet with much processed grains in the form of white flour or white rice, etc. which is low in the B vitamins in compared to a diet rich in whole grains.

The Common Ancient Human Diet

Humans have been hunter-gatherers since leaving the forests for life on the savanna 1.8 million years ago. Humans left the nomadic hunting-gathering lifestyle only about 10,000 years ago at the dawn of the agricultural age. From an evolutionary standpoint this is a very short period of time. Evolutionary changes in the body occur through natural selection and take much longer periods of time to emerge.

Our bodies are designed and equipped for eating the natural foods our ancestors consumed while living on the savanna (mainly vegetables, fruits, grains, seeds, underground storage organs, and legumes, and to a much lesser extent, lean red meat). Our bodies are designed and equipped to thrive with an active lifestyle and daily

Chapter 4 - Dietary Requirements: Comparison Between Apes and Humans

long distance walks like our ancient human ancestors did. They had great physical strength that allowed them to survive and reproduce through natural selection. They also lived past the age of seventy, if they survived childhood, and their deaths were mainly due to accidents and harsh weather conditions rather than to diseases.

In the previous chapter we explored the differences in digestive tract sizes between humans and gorillas and how early humans have physically changed throughout evolution and various survival methods. Let's recap and summarize this subject.

Our digestive tracts became smaller than those of gorillas due to the reduced need to digest cellulose-rich foods once grains were introduced into the diet. Our new and shortened digestive tract allowed more energy to be available to feed our growing brains which was needed to help us survive the harsh savanna and the constantly changing nomadic lifestyle. We looked at the difference between gorillas and hominins in the number of copies of the salivary amylase enzyme, responsible for the digestion of starches.

We saw duplication of the salivary amylase enzyme in early humans allowing them to consume grains, legumes and underground storage organs rich in carbohydrates, and use the energy stored in them as a regular source of energy to feed their larger and hungry brains and bodies without having to chew on and consume foods throughout the entire day.

And last, but not least, we are the only species who has learned to control fire and use it for cooking, making food more readily digestible and assailable.

These significant evolutionary changes gave us the edge over all other animals and allowed us to become the most sophisticated and advanced species on earth life form in the world today.

The growth of our brain to its current size happened many years before agriculture began. In fact, brain size has decreased since the dawn of agriculture. [198] In the past millennia, the average brain volume of Europeans was reduced from a previous mean value of 1502 ml to a recent value of 1241 ml. This decrease of approximately 240 ml in 10,000 years is nearly thirty-six times the rate of increase of brain volume during the previous 800,000 years. [198] Not only

Chapter 4 - Dietary Requirements: Comparison Between Apes and Humans

have we become more sedentary, we have also set about eating foods of much less variety and much less nutritional value. We eat high fat, sodium rich, processed foods that have been manufactured in factories instead of grown in nature, foods with artificial colorings and flavorings designed to make them look and taste sumptuous, but which have no relation to the natural, nutrient-dense foods we require to support our cells.

The knowledge and common sense as to what we need in order to thrive physically and mentally is unconsciously available in all of us. However, it is obscured by intensive brainwashing which we are exposed to through the media. It masks our natural intuition as to what is good for us and what is not. Today, all of the statistics and demographic information is readily available on the internet, but the simple and plain truths that I am providing you with throughout this book are not available in the media because natural foods and a natural lifestyle do not produce a profitable business.

This is where the equation of knowledge and self-empowerment comes into the picture. The more knowledge you have, the more power and control over your situation you will gain. The more you understand, the better position you will be in to care for yourself, your family, and to make educated life choices.

We have become so used to the comforts of modern living such as eating in restaurants, using microwaves to cook our foods, readymade meals, etc., all of which satisfy our taste buds and our clocks, but at the expense of our health. These unnatural foods and cooking methods help us to survive in the unnatural lifestyle settings we have created for ourselves that are a far cry from our natural way of living.

So what is natural for us to consume and how should we live in order to thrive?
Should we really be eating and living like our ancestors, the gorillas?

Well, the answer to that is yes and no. We should observe our physiological similarities and differences in order to understand what is the perfect diet for human consumption, and examine the right lifestyle choices that support human health based on human

Chapter 4 - Dietary Requirements: Comparison Between Apes and Humans

evolution, our genes, and on the latest technological advances in all of the scientific fields.

Technology has come such a long way in the past century with the best human minds creating outstanding feats and discoveries in all fields, including the medical field, which has helped save many lives. We can see how far we have advanced just looking around us and seeing an amazing array of incredible things we don't usually pay any detailed attention to because we have become so accustomed to having them in our lives. But, on the other hand, mounting evidence suggests that it is by going back to our true natural diet, the diet of early humans and previous species in our genus, while employing the technological discoveries that are now available to us in all scientific fields, we can achieve ideal health and the longevity we seek as well as reach even more outstanding feats with the brains we have developed.

The Diet Best Suited for Human Consumption

In recent years there is mounting evidence that the best diet for human consumption is a natural, mainly plant-based, whole food diet with small amounts of lean meat peppered in to add vitamin B12. There is also mounting evidence that shows that this was the original diet our ancestors consumed.

During the Stone Age, as hunter-gatherers, humans were foraging for food, wandering around in a nomadic lifestyle, selecting the foods and plants they wanted to eat. Their foods grew naturally in their habitat and were freely available for immediate consumption. There was no food storage. Fresh foods were consumed daily and directly from the plants on which they grew. Most foods were consumed in their natural states.

The diet of the earliest hominins included large quantities of fruit, leaves, wild berries, roots, leafy vegetables, vegetable shoots, wild grains, flowers, underground storage organs, legumes, and water with some insects, [199, 200] and small quantities of raw meat.

Chapter 4 - Dietary Requirements: Comparison Between Apes and Humans

Studies of tooth morphology suggest that the diet of hominins also included hard food items such as seeds and nuts, roots, and tubers. [201, 202, 203] The teeth of humans before the dawn of agriculture were stronger and healthier than those of humans after agriculture began. [204, 205, 206] Research shows that humans come from a plant eating lineage and obtained the bulk of their diets from plant foods. [207] This is perhaps why a plant-based diet is most suitable for humans. Although our gut has become slightly smaller, as well as our bodies, our brains have grown bigger since this time. Anatomically, not much else has changed since the time of *Homo erectus*, dating from around 1.85 million years ago [208] after the hominin species became erect, left the rain forests, and learned to survive on the African savanna. Cooking was only introduced much later, around 300,000 years ago. This had further influence on our brain size which by then tripled in size compared to our early ancestor's brains, from 350 cm^3 in volume to 1250 cm^3 in volume in present day humans. We further see a major increase in capabilities about 60,000 years ago, after speech was introduced through a genetic change.

Brain growth was not due to agriculture which only really took off 8,000 years ago. [209]

Our brains developed and made serious progress during the time when we fed mostly on plant foods, grains, legumes, underground storage organs, and a little meat when available. Hominins only began consuming fish in those populations who left Africa about 40,000 years ago, but the populations who remained in Africa did not rely on fish as a regular food source and only sparingly on meat since they had many natural crops easily available for them to eat. However, many human populations who left Africa and scattered around the world did live near shores allowing humans to consume marine animals that were in abundance and were not dangerous to humans. The roles and effects of meat and fish consumption are covered in detail in Chapter 6.

Chapter 4 - Dietary Requirements: Comparison Between Apes and Humans

The Dawn of Agriculture and the Modern Human Diet

Agriculture began simultaneously in two places on the globe 12,000 years ago. One is an area east of the Mediterranean known as the *"fertile crescent,"* which is characterized by an abundance of naturally growing grains, fruit trees, and shrubs. This area runs from Israel to Syria and into Iraq. At the same time agriculture began to form around the Nile in Egypt. Both areas are part of the geographic corridor through which humans moved through when leaving Africa. Agriculture began gradually, through casual cultivation, to help expanding families sustain themselves more easily without moving frequently, which further enhanced the growth of the families.

About 8,000 years ago agriculture appeared in other places as well, beginning in Eurasia, but only around 4,000 years ago do we see agriculture becoming globally widespread and reaching the Americas.

How did it happen that places so far away from each other began to farm land at around the same time although there was no apparent contact between them? Scientists think that two factors were involved: Weather conditions that supported this agricultural age, and a growing population which forced people to increase the availability of their food sources.

1. **Global Weather Conditions Change to Support Agriculture:** Global climate gradually became warmer and the ice sheets of the last glacial period melted. Rivers were formed, oceans expanded, and the weather became wetter and more predictable than during the Ice Age. In the Ice Age rocks degraded into mineral dust that spread with winds and enriched the soil. Trees and food were everywhere 12,000 years ago. The warming and more regular weather patterns formed the perfect setting for the dawn of agriculture. Resources such as plants and animals became more abundant and this allowed populations of humans to become less nomadic. They could fulfil their dietary needs quite easily by staying in one place. Once they had

abundant resources, they also felt secure enough to reproduce more often than they had in the past.

2. **The Population Grows Leaving People with No Choice But to Grow Their Own Food:** The population began to grow and villages began to appear. The expanding population around the world meant that there were less free land areas to move into once resources in a specific land area were exhausted.

At the dawn of the Neolithic era approximately 10,000 years ago, there is evidence that the global human population was between 1 - 4 million people. About 8000 years ago, after agriculture appeared around the world, the global population was approximately 5 million. Over the next 7,000 year period, up to 1 A.D., the population grew at a rate of 0.05% per year and global population reached 200 million. [210] This increase in population was made possible through agriculture which allowed us to grow and raise our own foods to feed and sustain a whole community for a long period of time.

People began to reproduce at much higher rates than they did when they were hunter-gatherers because there was no need to carry small children from place to place as often as they had done previously, thereby making life easier. [211] As they reproduced, their communities expanded until they could not continue the nomadic way of life. The lands around them were now inhabited by other growing communities. This population increase led to further domestication of many more crops. With time, all of the continents on the globe became populated, each with its own expanding population, so people had to make the most of the land on which they lived. Families remained on one plot of land and built houses for themselves, while the skills needed to forage were slowly lost as new generations were brought up into the agricultural society.

Agriculture is very different from foraging for food. Only specific plants were selected for domestication, mainly those which were the easiest to cultivate, the tastiest, and most beautiful. Ancient agriculture was developed by trial and error. What grew easily was

Chapter 4 - Dietary Requirements: Comparison Between Apes and Humans

used; what was not easy to grow or did not yield enough produce was discarded.

Slowly a dependency formed: domesticated plants and animals became dependent on humans for their existence, and humans, with an ever expanding population, became dependent on those domesticated animals and plants for their survival. This interdependence sometimes led to selection of crops which was contrary to the evolutionary process, where crops that would not have survived naturally were selected for their genetic mutations such as bananas without seeds, olives with high oil content and non-popping peas. [212] Later fruit trees were cultivated by a complex technique called grafting, first developed in China, whereby tissues from one plant were mounted on another plant so that the two sets of tissues join together in asexual propagation.

The Introduction of Fertilizers

Plants depend on nutrients found in the soil for their nutrient requirements. The supply of these components in the soil is limited, and as plants were grown over and over in the same soils, they used up the soils nutrients. Therefore the availability of these nutrients in the soil gradually decreased with each harvest, causing a reduction in the quality and yield of the crops.

People then created fertilizers — substances that are added to the soil to improve the plants growth and yield. These fertilizers helped replace the natural nutrients that were used up by the cultivated crops.

The process of fertilizing the land by adding substances to the soil in order to improve its fertility was developed during the earliest days of agriculture. Farmers found out that the yield could be improved by spreading animal manure on the soil. This was the first use of fertilizers.

Over time, fertilizers were improved and new substances that increased the yield were developed. The Egyptians added ashes from burned weeds. [213] Ancient Greek and Roman writings indicate that various animal excrements were used, depending on the type of soil or plant grown. [213] It was also known by this time that growing leguminous plants on plots prior to growing wheat was beneficial to increasing yield. Other substances were added to soils including seashells, clay, vegetable and waste from different manufacturing processes.

As the nutritional needs of plants were discovered and understood, fertilizer technology advanced.

The effects of fertilizers and later the development of pesticides on health will be examined in the next chapter, but for now let me state that it is evident that bacteria, crop diseases, and weeds are inherent in agriculture, and if insecticides and fertilizers were not available, entire crops could be wiped out and the stability of our current food supply would be shaken. Food supply would decrease, resulting in major food price increases. [213] Using fertilizers and pesticides became (almost) the only way to feed the large population we currently have on earth.

The Introduction Of Domesticated Animals For Meat

The first domesticated animals to be used for meat as a food source were mouflons that were domesticated into modern sheep. Wild boars then became domesticated farm pigs, and aurochs became domesticated cows which were used for meat. [214] At first keeping domesticated animals required moving around a lot since the herds always needed fresh grass to feed on. Over time, humans used agriculture to change the diets of domesticated animals into grains instead of grasses, which were grown to feed humans as well as animals about 3,000 years ago. At first this seemed like a perfect solution and it was adapted by almost all human communities globally. However, there were many consequences to the domestication of animals that were not recognized at the time.

The introduction of domesticated animals for meat resulted in increased meat consumption, far beyond what had previously been consumed in hunter-gatherer societies. These societies ate meat sparsely, according to availability, and it is estimated that less than

15% of the hunting expeditions were successful. (See Chapter 3 for detailed discussion of meat as an ancient food source.)

Alison Brooks, a paleoanthropologist from George Washington University, says: "According to the evidence no one ate meat all that often, except in the Arctic." (215)

Was Agriculture a Healthier Way of Life? Did Agriculture Improve Human Health?

Professor Jared Diamond, an American scientist who received the prestigious Wolf Prize in Agriculture in 2013, thinks not. He states that: "The average height of hunter-gatherers toward the end of the Ice Ages was a generous 5' 9" (180 cm) for men, 5' 5" (167 cm) for women. However, with the adoption of agriculture, height diminished, and by 3000 B. C. had reached a low of only 5' 3" (162 cm) for men, 5' (152 cm) for women." Furthermore, he states that when comparing hunter-gatherer societies that preceded agriculture "The agricultural farmers' (remains) had a nearly 50% increase in enamel defects indicative of malnutrition, a fourfold increase in iron-deficiency anemia (evidenced by a bone condition called porotic hyperostosis), a threefold rise in bone lesions reflecting infectious disease in general, and an increase in degenerative conditions of the spine, probably reflecting a lot of hard physical labor." (204, 205, 206)

Humans paid a hefty price to allow for a growing population, including periods of starvation, the rise of infectious diseases, as well as conflicts, oppression, and slavery.

The Introduction of the Sedentary Lifestyle

As foragers in the pre-agriculture eras, humans had free time to create tools, art, jewellery, and to migrate. They were foraging for food only to fulfil their own and their family's needs, and were expending energy while foraging for food. When agriculture was introduced, aside from the farmers themselves, most humans became more sedentary by creating a more controllable food supply, and also by creating food in surplus which allowed people not directly involved in the collection/production of food to be supported by physically hard working farmers.

The Advantages and Disadvantages of Agriculture

Agriculture did indeed lead to a massive increase in population size by allowing permanent human settlements and the world's first communities to evolve, which relied on the surplus of food available to feed more mouths. However, it is important to look into the disadvantages as well as the advantages of agriculture when examining the ideal diet for human consumption. I'm referring to the best human diet that will ensure good health and longevity for the individual as well as support the sustainability of our globe.

The dawn of agriculture was marked by increased security of food availability in exchange for hard labor. Since then agriculture has come a long way over the last 10,000 years. It has allowed humans to populate and build civilizations in almost all corners of the globe. In the beginnings of agriculture, people did not need to leave their homes to go to work as we do today. Instead they worked their own land.

For thousands of years farmers lived a simple life without modern-day technology. Their lives were peaceful, but not easy. People had a lower life expectancy in comparison with previous hunter-gatherers due to malnutrition from poor food variation and poor living conditions. [204, 205, 206]

The global population continued to increase and by the year 1720 the global population reached 600 million.

However, modern day agriculture is not the natural growth of food as it started out to be. Today, following the industrial revolution which began in the late 1700s, agriculture is driven by fossil fuels, synthetic fertilizers, and toxic pesticides, as well as hormones and medicines used in the breeding of farm animals, resulting in food products that are often contaminated, unhealthy,

Chapter 4 - Dietary Requirements: Comparison Between Apes and Humans

and creating a huge environmental burden. Following the industrial revolution, the population doubled and reached 1.2 billion people in the early 1800's. [216, 217]

Human population reached the three billion mark less than thirty years after the second billion mark was reached in 1959. The fourth billion mark was then reached only fifteen years later in 1974, and the fifth billion in only thirteen years, in 1987.

During the 20th century alone, the population in the world has grown from 1.65 billion to 6 billion! In 1970, there were roughly half as many people in the world as there are now.

The world population reached the 7 billion mark in 2011. [218] In the latest United Nations projections, the global population will grow and stabilize at just above 10 billion persons after 2062. [219]

Society as we know it would not have developed without the use of fossil fuels which are part of all modern day fertilizers and pesticides, and are an integral part of everyday life as we know it. In fact, the use of fossil fuels is what allowed populations to grow immensely.

Modern agriculture is unbelievably dependent on fossil fuels, much more than we realize.

Firstly, agriculture requires gasoline and/or diesel to operate the machinery that plows the land and plants the seeds.

Secondly, there is the need for energy to irrigate, protect (using fungicides, insecticides, and herbicides all made from fossil fuels), and fertilize the crops (made from natural gas).

Thirdly, more machines using some type of fossil fuel come into play during the harvesting and drying of the crops.

Later the crops are driven, using fuel again, to big industrial plants to be processed.

Lastly, crops are flown, driven, or shipped via cargo boats to the place where they are sold. All of these modes of transport use fossil fuels to power.

Meat production is another fossil fuel greedy industry. Domesticated animals eat a lot of grain if they do not have pastures to roam freely in and feed on grasses. For example, one cow eats about half a ton of grain per year. That's about 54,000 calories from

Chapter 4 - Dietary Requirements: Comparison Between Apes and Humans

grain per day for each cow, in comparison to 2000 calories required on average to feed a person per day. The extensive use of fossil fuels and deforestation practices used to clear land for the purpose of raising meat for food has become a major burden on the environment.

The Effects of Modern Agriculture on Human Behavior and Society

Human behavior changed as a result of agriculture.

Due to the promise of monetary reward of high yields, humans learned to protect their crops and animals. They learned to protect their land and animals by diverting rivers and building dams. People became greedy and began clearing forests to allow more space for fields to grow more crops, or to raise livestock for their own personal monetary benefit.

Fossil fuel wells and mines were created everywhere for people to get their hands on fossil fuels for monetary gains. Pesticides were created to kill pests that harmed crops, and cheaper chemical fertilizers were used to create larger yields.

Social classes were formed and land became harder to get.

However, we must look at reality as it is and not as we would like it to be. The situation today is that we are dependent on agriculture for our food whether we like it or not. But one thing is certain: agriculture systems need to be transformed if we are to sustain the future population and the health of the people as well as our earth.

Modern day agriculture is not sustainable, neither for human health nor for the health of our planet.

It's no coincidence that the quest for the best human diet should also lead us towards a more natural, environmentally sustainable and animal friendly food production line.

Chapter 4 - Dietary Requirements: Comparison Between Apes and Humans

We are currently using 10 calories of fossil fuel energy for every 1 calorie of food we eat. This way of life is fundamentally unsustainable and cannot continue due to the effect on the Earth's capacity to withstand the harmful byproducts of fossil fuel combustion.

To sustain the population of 10+ billion people, we need to begin transforming the agriculture systems and the food choices we are making today.

In the next chapter we shall go over human health with an evolutionary and comparative perspective.

Chapter 5

Human Health – Ancient Times vs. Modern Times

"Let food be thy medicine and medicine be thy food."

– Hippocrates

There have been huge advances in modern agriculture and medicine through scientific research. However, we see growing numbers of sick people suffering from degenerative and chronic diseases. Have our advances led us in the right direction towards health and longevity of our species, and if not, can we do anything about it?

Modern agriculture has shown us the way to producing pretty foods in surplus; however, there are still populations on earth that are suffering from malnutrition. On the other hand, there are other populations that are suffering the consequences of excess nutrition leading to obesity. Medical research has allowed us to overcome many infectious diseases providing almost all children born today with the ability to live a long life. But what about our quality of life?

Modern agriculture has led to our dependence on fossil fuels for food. These fossil fuels have a degenerative effect on our environment. Our fields are starving from mineral depletion and our foods are suffering from low nutrient levels due to the modern, unnatural cultivation of the land.

Chapter 5 - Human Health – Ancient Times vs. Modern Times

Foods are grown to make the consumers happy with foods produced to look nice irrelevant of their nutritional status.

Agriculture has found ways to provide foods out of season by growing them in energy expensive greenhouses for higher profits. People are willing to pay much money for foods that are ripened even one month before their natural season arrives. Foods that are less pretty are not likely to be bought by consumers shopping in supermarkets simply because foods that are prettier are placed right beside them in supermarket aisles. But to make produce look so nice, it is covered with waxes, and washed and sprayed with chemicals after it has left the field before it even reaches the supermarket shelves. By consuming only attractive foods, perfectly round and shiny, not wrinkled or withered, we are forcing farmers to produce foods that are not real and certainly not natural. The energy cost for this production and the cost to the globe and to our personal health is tremendous.

We, as consumers, have an effect on this through what we choose to consume, hence affecting the health of our globe and our own personal health.

Nowadays we are becoming aware of various disorders in Western societies that are not observed in modern hunter-gatherer populations. [220, 221] This has led a number of researchers, including myself, to conclude that humans have not really adapted to diets of domesticated, genetically modified, processed plant and animal foods common in Western societies today. [222, 223, 224] As mentioned in the previous chapter, these foods are considered recent on an evolutionary timescale. Furthermore, the variation of our foods has declined in comparison to hunter-gatherer pre-agricultural populations.

As I have pointed out in the previous chapter, evidence shows that there is a general decrease in body stature, tooth size, and an increase in dental cavities after the dawn of the agricultural age. The smaller teeth we see in modern humans are due to the consumption of easier to chew processed foods like breads and porridges. The simple carbohydrate contents of these foods results in the increased dental problems common in Western societies, as well as a whole range of diseases associated with the consumption of processed foods and the sedentary and urbanized lifestyle that followed the increased reliance on domesticated foods through agriculture. (225)

To allow for such a dramatic increase in human population size, food production increased beyond the capacity of the environment. The trade off our ancestors made for major population growth was a declined personal and global health state.

However, the tradeoff of a general decline in individual health and environmental health we made thousands of years ago need not proceed today. (226)

By examining how culture, rather than genetics, has affected our health, we can also look toward a way of life that will help us remain healthy to a much older age; one that will also have the same positive influence on the future generations of our children, grandchildren, and even further down the line, as well as on our planet at large. Choices that we make today will have consequences way into the future, so by making thoughtful, well researched decisions we can support long term human health and happiness as well as the health of the world at large.

Ancient Human Health and Life Expectancy (Before Agriculture)

What was the life expectancy of *Homo Ergaster*, *Homo Erectus*, and early *Homo sapiens*?

Before the dawn of agriculture, life expectancy was actually longer for humans than it was after the dawn of agriculture between 10,000 years ago up until 200 years ago, where we see a serious drop in life expectancy, only to have it rise again in the last two centuries.

In the early Stone Age, which lasted from about 2.6 million to approximately 300,000 years ago when cooking began, (227) it is estimated that a person who managed to survive up until the age of fifteen years had the life expectancy of seventy-four to eighty years. (228)

Chapter 5 - Human Health – Ancient Times vs. Modern Times

While we lack any concrete data for infant and child mortality rates in such early populations, we may estimate them by using those found in modern hunter-gatherer societies. I do realize that using "modern" hunter-gatherer group data to infer on rates in the past is filled with potential problems. Modern groups are not perfect replicas of ancient groups due to the possible exposure to modern sanitation and medicine, thereby reducing originality and the possibility to conduct a fair comparison between modern hunter-gatherers and prehistoric ones. [229] Furthermore, ancient hunter-gatherer lives are mainly based on written descriptions by explorers, military personnel, missionaries, colonial officials, naturalists, ethnologists, and behavioral ecologists, who met them and may have been biased with their own opinions. Thus ancient mortality rates remain educated estimates. However, scientists found that once infant mortality rates were removed, early humans had the same life expectancy as found in present day modern societies, [230, 231] and according to fossil records, early humans tended to die from accidents and external injuries rather than from diseases as we see in modern society.

On the other hand, if mortality rates of children are not removed from the equation, and half of all children died by age twelve, then the average life expectancy would be forty, because life expectancy is an average of everyone. This means that if half of the children died before the age of twelve (at the average age of death of six years), for the life expectancy at birth to come out to be forty then the remaining half would be expected to live on average up to the age of seventy-four, with the consequence that roughly a quarter of all babies born would live to be older than seventy-four.

In present-day hunter-gatherer tribes, most individuals survive after childhood, and the same can be concluded for human populations 50,000 years ago. [232] However, during all historical times, except in modern times, childhood has been associated with the highest levels of mortality. [233]

Chapter 5 - Human Health – Ancient Times vs. Modern Times

Neolithic Human Health and Life Expectancy (At the Dawn of Agriculture)

After the beginning of agriculture, around 10,000 years ago, during the Neolithic era, life expectancy dropped to twenty years, and for those surviving up to the age of ten years, life expectancy was then only an additional thirty-five to thirty-seven years (to bring the total life expectancy age to between forty-five and forty-seven years). [234] But why did life expectancy decrease so much during this period?

There are a few reasons to explain this drop.

Firstly, man's eating habits changed dramatically. Animal breeding allowed him to consume meat on a regular basis, although not exactly the same kind of meat as he was eating during the previous hunter-gatherer period which were very lean pieces of meat from animals surviving naturally in nature. Domesticated animals have higher fat levels partly due to their sedentary nature.

The development of agriculture allowed man to plant his own food. But farmers considerably reduced the variety of the foods they ate from the time they were hunter-gatherers and only certain crops were grown. This tendency to grow one sole crop, normally a staple one, exposed farmers to much risk. When harvests were poor, the effects became disastrous. Furthermore, growing a sole staple crop led people to suffer from nutrient deficiencies leading to a shortened life span.

One would have imagined that agriculture would have brought about an improvement in man's existence, but, as we can see, this was certainly not the case at the time.

When man made the decision to start controlling his own food sources and stop migrating from place to place, he came across new difficulties. Farming the land was much more physically demanding than hunting and gathering for food. The soil needed to be irrigated regularly, plowed, and then the food required harvesting. Man was forced to face unstable weather conditions; he had to choose less fragile plant varieties to grow on not so perfect soils and only specific animal species to raise. This lowered the variety of foods and thereby nutrients man had available to eat.

The population grew, but life span shortened during this period.

Modern Day Human Health and Life Expectancy

In 1900, global average life expectancy was just thirty-one years, and below fifty years even in the richest countries. But by the mid-20th century, average life expectancy rose to forty-eight years.

In 2005, average lifespan reached 65.6 years, and over 80 years in some countries. [235]

Over the period 2010–2015, the average human life expectancy at birth was 72 years (69.2 years for males and 75 years for females). [236] It is interesting to see how life expectancy increased over the past sixty-five years in the chart below

Table 2. Global life expectancy at birth for both sexes (yrs)

1950-1955	1955-1960	1960-1965	1965-1970	1970-1975	1975-1980	1980-1985	1985-1990	1990-1995	1995-2000	2000-2005	2005-2010	2010-2015
47	49	51	57	59	61	62	64	65	66	67	69	72

The infant mortality rate for 2011 was 6.5 infant deaths per thousand live births. Infant mortality rate has statistically remained the same or decreased significantly each successive year from 1958 through 2011. [237, 238]

Modern medicine and public health measures are allowing people to live longer. Childhood mortality rates are now reduced to a level as low as 1%.

But has the quality of life increased with the increase in lifespan?

Let's have a look at the leading causes of death.

Chapter 5 - Human Health – Ancient Times vs. Modern Times

Today, the leading causes of death in the world today are as follows: [239, 240]

1. Heart disease: with 17.3 million global deaths each year. This number is expected to rise to more than 23.6 million global deaths from heart disease by 2030. [240]
2. Stroke (CVA, TIA): The number of people having first and recurrent strokes each year went up, reaching 33 million in 2010.
3. Cancer
4. Chronic lower respiratory diseases
5. Accidents
6. Alzheimer's disease
7. Diabetes
8. Influenza and Pneumonia
9. Kidney diseases
10. Suicide

It seems that although lifespan has increased, quality of life has not. Although the majority of people may look rather healthy, statistics show a different story. Nearly 1 in 2 Americans (133 million) [241] is suffering from a chronic disease which have many implications on the quality of their lives today. [242] Sixty percent of adults up to the age of 64 years are suffering from a chronic disease and this number goes up to 90% for seniors. [243]

Modern human advances in medicine and technology during the past few decades generated a transition in society with rapidly increasing numbers of middle-aged and elderly people. A new set of diseases rose including cancers, heart disease, stroke, and mental illness, with less satisfying results from medications than we achieved for infectious diseases through the invention of antibiotics.

In this era there is no option for a quick pill or medicine to help save our health. It is only through the changing of our hardwired lifestyle choices and return to a more in tune with nature approach to health that we can increase quality of life and increase life expectancy even more.

Chapter 5 - Human Health – Ancient Times vs. Modern Times

Actually, by observing the common modern human diet, it is quite amazing that we have such long life spans when two of the top five sources of calories in the modern Western world diet are sugars, including sugary drinks, cakes, cookies, pies, and pastries. Both food sources contribute calories, but do not offer any nutritional value. When it comes to meat consumption throughout the world, Americans come in second to Luxembourg, averaging 270 pounds per person per year. [244] Both meat and poultry are a major source of saturated fat. High intakes of saturated fat raise blood cholesterol levels and the raise the risk of heart disease and stroke, two of the five leading causes of death in the Western world.

When it comes to food choices, in the modern Western society, convenience plays a major role. Convenience foods include meals eaten out and foods purchased at the grocery store that help make home meal preparation faster and easier. Convenience foods tend to be high in saturated fat, salt, and added sugar, and they offer very little nutritional value.

In fact, research shows that poor lifestyle behaviors and poor food choices are "the foremost causes of death and disability in the United States and in the world" as stated by The American Heart Association in their 2015 update of heart disease and stroke statistics. [245]

Farming created surpluses of food, [246] and processing of foods, especially grains and sugar, helped drastically extend their storage period. Processing also allowed for easy measurement as well as long distance transportation due to their small size, hardiness, and dryness of these processed products. [247]

Nowadays, almost all food types are easily and cheaply attainable everywhere in the Western world with almost no physical effort on our part due to modern transportation. It is through the easy attainability of foods, requiring almost no energy output, and the almost endless variety of unnatural and convenient foods available on all parts of the globe which has offered us a lazy approach to feeding ourselves, and this has given us most of our modern day health problems.

Chapter 5 - Human Health – Ancient Times vs. Modern Times

It is obvious that living in comfort with air conditioned or heated houses with sanitation at our disposal have increased the quality of our lives dramatically. Buying our foods at the local grocery has also increased our livelihood. This extra free time has allowed us humans to spend it doing other, more creative activities to further improve the world around us. However, not all of us use this time creatively. Some people find themselves often sitting in front of the television set or doing some other sedentary, mind dulling activity while feeding their bodies with highly processed, high energy comfort foods without even noticing what they are doing. Thus we are exerting less physical energy for food collection, and the foods consumed tend to be richer in calories and lacking in nutrients. Muscular strength is reduced due to a decrease in fitness levels, leaving us with epidemics like obesity, diabetes, and heart disease which arise from lowered insulin sensitivity, lowered metabolism, increased fat in our body composition, and a chronic state of inflammation. These diseases were rare to non-existent among primitive humans. [248] Dietary habits and physical activity levels play an essential role in the development of these diseases. [249, 250]

Humans evolved from being active nomad food foragers who expended enormous amounts of energy on a daily basis, not only due to immense physical demands in the search of food, but also because living conditions were extremely precarious, particularly due to the unpredictable weather conditions.

Early humans had to expend energy in order to maintain their body temperature and also to eat. Nowadays there is hardly any energy expended during the collection of foods. [251] In short, agriculture bred immobility and we began suffering from a chronic state of disease reducing the quality of our lives immensely.

So how do we change this situation?

Only by changing what we eat will we be able to change and improve our own destiny as well as that of our future generations and of our planet Earth.

In the next chapters we shall go into the principles of *The Guerrilla Diet and Lifestyle Program* and the reasons behind them.

Chapter 6

The Theory Behind Reducing Meat Products in Your Diet

"The cow eats three basic things in their feed: corn, beets, and barley, and so what I do is I actually challenge my staff with these crazy, wild ideas. Can we take what the cow eats, remove the cow, and then make some hamburgers out of that?"

— Homaro Cantu

We are told constantly of the high nutritional value of meat products. We constantly hear in the media about the necessity of consuming meat for protein, and the especially important role of meat for children. People are actually choosing kindergartens by the amount of meat served per week for their children. But is this belief really true? Does meat play such an important role in human nutrition? Is consuming meat so important for our health? All of these questions will be answered in this chapter.

At first it was assumed that humans incorporated meat into their diet and this is what allowed our brains to grow to be incredibly large when compared to our body size. [252] As discussed in chapter 3, brain growth in the *Homo* lineage began about 2 million years ago.

Chapter 6 - The Theory Behind Reducing Meat Products in Your Diet

Brain growth was so advantageous for hominin survival on the savanna to warrant the use of so much energy to fuel it. The brain required a regular and stable food source to support its growth. The regular, stable food source that supported brain growth to take on such a large size in comparison with total body weight was not meat, but rather legumes and grains found in plentitude on the savanna and grasslands where hominins evolved.

If we really look into the history of human kind we will find that the role of plant foods had a prominent role throughout all early human diets, [253, 254] until the time of agriculture when plants became domesticated for food about 10,000 years ago and animals become widely domesticated for food 4,000 years ago. The domestication of animals for food led to a very significant increase in meat consumption which began only around 3,000 years ago. This represents less than 0.002% of the human history if we examine our evolution since we departed from the apes 6 million years ago, and 0.003% of our time on earth if we look back at the time of *Homo erectus*, 1.85 million years ago, when our brains began to expand.

Dental calculus, a form of hardened dental plaque, is increasingly recognized as a major reservoir of dietary information. Amanda Henry an American Paleoanthropologist has been examining fossil dental calculus with her team at Leipzig University. They found that plant matter had an important role in the human diet even at the time of Neanderthals 400,000 years ago. Henry examines data from the analysis of plant micro-remains (starch grains and fossilized particles of plant tissue) in dental calculus and on ancient stone tools. Her results suggested that Neanderthals consumed a wide array of plant foods, including underground storage organs and grass seeds. Plant matter and starch grains recovered from dental calculus were found to be consumed by the entire range of ancient individuals found in the sites they examined, including Shanidar Cave in Iraq, and Spy Cave in Belgium. None of the expected predictors of variation (species, geographic region, or associated stone tool technology) had a strong influence on the number of plant species consumed. [255] Some of the plants are typical of recent modern human diets, including date palms, legumes, and

Chapter 6 - The Theory Behind Reducing Meat Products in Your Diet

grass seeds, whereas others are known to be edible but are not heavily consumed today. In later fossils, the team of scientists found that many of the grass seed starches showed damage that is a distinctive marker of cooking. Their results indicate that in both warm eastern Mediterranean and cold north-western European climates, and across their latitudinal range, Neanderthals made use of the diverse plant foods available in their local environment and transformed them into more easily digestible foodstuffs in part through cooking them. [256] This evidence shows that plant foods were a major contributor in Neanderthal dietary regimes from as early as 400,000 years ago up until as late as 30,000 years ago when Neanderthals disappeared from the fossil record.

More research studies also show that plant foods had a more prominent role in early human diets. [257, 258, 259, 260, 261]

Furthermore, studies of existing hunter-gatherers have shown that vegetable foods comprised a larger percentage of early human diets than did meat.

As of yet there is no research that can show the quantity of grain and plant foods in these early human diets, but a major research project I mentioned in chapter 3 called *The Lost Crops Of Africa*, [262] suggests that gathering grains from Africa's Savannah "is among the most sustainable organized food production systems in the world. It was common in the Stone Age and has been important almost ever since, especially in Africa's drylands. For millennia people living in and about the Sahara gathered grass seeds on a grand scale." [262]

It was wild grains such as wheat and barley grasses, millet, and African rice along with carbohydrate rich underground storage organs that were the high quality foods found on the African Savannah that allowed us to grow our energy expensive brains and to slowly evolve into the highly developed species we are today.

Meat was not the food that allowed this to happen.

Chapter 6 - The Theory Behind Reducing Meat Products in Your Diet

When Did Our Awe For Meat Protein Begin?

It began in the early 1900s when food supply was sufficient to provide the energy (calories) people needed, but foods were lacking in protein due to the processing they went through before consumption.

As the industrial revolution spread and food processing became popular for storage and transport purposes, grass grains that could originally supply a wealth of nutrients, including protein, were stripped of their healthy germ layer and made into processed white wheat that had the ability to be stored for years without rotting, could easily be transported, and supplied energy in the form of calories, but, on the other hand, supplied little nutritional value. The whole grain unprocessed version would rot quite quickly in comparison to the stripped white version, and could not be stored for long periods before refrigeration was discovered. This caused large populations, who were dependent on grains and who processed them as well, to develop protein deficiency. This led to the discovery of a disease later called Kwashiorkor by the Jamaican pediatrician, Cicely Williams, who introduced the name into the medical community in her 1935 Lancet article. [263] This disease came from a severe protein-energy malnutrition characterized by bloating, irritability, and a fatty, enlarged liver. [264] Kwashiorkor mainly affected small children whom were weaned from breast milk too soon and moved on to consume processed grains instead. Cicely Williams corrected their nutritional protein deficiency by supplementing their diet with protein and these children regained their health. The World Health Organization took these findings very seriously and declared protein deficiency as a world crisis. Research groups at the time were receiving generous government funding to find a solution to protein malnutrition.

In the mid-1960s, Professor T. Colin Campbell, a nutritional biochemist, was sent by the US State Department for International Development to the Philippines with an agenda to end childhood malnutrition by getting more high quality protein into their diets. Campbell, while in the Philippines, searched for a locally produced,

Chapter 6 - The Theory Behind Reducing Meat Products in Your Diet

inexpensive, high protein source. As a nutritionist at the time, protein had become the main focus for research and his findings from the Philippines would *shake his view* on the subject completely. His findings clearly showed that the children who ate the most protein rich diets were actually most likely to suffer from liver cancer when compared to children who had lower protein consumption. [265]

In fact, if it were true that we needed such high protein diets to thrive, then certainly gorillas and the other apes would also be eating protein in high quantities, but this was not the case. In fact, a gorilla's diet in the wild consists of foods very low in fat and protein in comparison to their total daily caloric intake, about 10%.

If humans would have turned to meat as a source of protein due to lack of protein in their diet, it is probable that we would have seen gorillas and chimpanzees, our closest living relatives who share 98% to 99% of our genes, do the same, [266] but we do not see this happening. Gorillas have remained 98% vegan throughout evolution and chimpanzees are 94% vegan. Gorillas and chimpanzees get only a very small portion of their diet from animal protein and they rarely, if ever, scavenge for meat [267], most likely because they cannot efficiently digest raw meat. [268]

Through the years and the many research projects and epidemiological studies done on the human diet, we can see that protein shortage was never a serious problem for primates nor for humans until grain processing began. There is no need for "high-quality" protein sources such as those that come from animal products to maintain our health. Humans, like gorillas and other great apes, require 8 essential amino acids from the diet out of the 20 amino acids needed to build proteins. Essential amino acids must be supplied by the diet because the body cannot create them, unlike the remaining 12 amino acids which are not essential and can be made in the body. We require protein in the diet because within our bodies proteins wear down regularly and new proteins are constantly being synthesized to replace depleted ones as well as those lost during stages of growth. The protein ingested is broken down into individual amino acids and then put back together again as new protein in a process called protein biosynthesis. The entire amino acid pool

Chapter 6 - The Theory Behind Reducing Meat Products in Your Diet

changes three to four times a day. Proteins take part in many of the body's basic functions including:
- Enzyme production which catalyze chemical reactions in the body
- Hormone production involved in regulatory processes
- Transport protein production which carries various substances to and from body tissues and in and out of the cells
- Lipoprotein production which transport fat and cholesterol around the body
- Antibody production which play an important role in healthy immune function
- Maintenance of a normal acid-base balance
- Maintenance of proper fluid balance in and out of the cells
- As well as in structural proteins which make up muscle tissue, connective tissue, hair, nails, and skin.

The 8 essential amino acids include: Isoleucine, Lysine, Leucine, Methionine, Phenylalanine, Threonine, Tryptophan, Valine, and Arginine, and are all found in both animal and vegetable proteins.

However, research shows that it is **less** important and even less beneficial to receive all of these amino acids from one "high-quality protein" source, such as those from animal proteins. [269, 270, 271] It *is* necessary for both gorillas and humans to have a diet with sufficient amino acids to meet protein requirements, but there is no need for high quality forms of protein because it is through slow and steady synthesis of new proteins from "low quality" plant proteins that has proven to be healthier for humans. [272]

If the body is deficient in essential amino acids from dietary sources, the body is not able to build proteins and will have to break down muscle tissue to obtain the essential amino acids it requires. On a natural diet with varied plant sources, the goal of incorporating all of the essential amino acids in the diet is easily achieved.

A Comparison Between Human Breast Milk and Other Mammal Milk Composition

It is wise also to look at human breast milk of lactating women to determine how much protein humans really need. The protein content of human breast milk is actually the lowest in comparison with other lactating mammals. Milk from cows and goats is much higher in protein, calcium, and sodium, and much lower in mono and polyunsaturated fats, carbohydrates, folate, and vitamin C in comparison to human milk.

Table 3: A Comparison Between Mammal Milk Compositions

Nutrients	**Human Milk**	**Cow Milk**	**Goat Milk**
Calories	172	146	168
Protein (g)	2.5	7.9	8.7
Fat (g)	10.8	7.9	10.1
Saturated fat (g)	4.9	4.6	6.5
Monounsat-urated fat (g)	4.1	2.0	2.7
Polyunsaturated fat (g)	1.2	0.5	0.4
Carbohydrate (g)	17.0	11.0	10.9
Folate (mcg)	12	12	2
Vitamin C (mg)	12.3	0	3.2
Sodium (mg)	42	98	122
Iron (mg)	0.07	0.07	0.12
Calcium (mg)	79	276	327

Source: U.S. Department of Agriculture, Agricultural Research Service. 2004. [273]

Chapter 6 - The Theory Behind Reducing Meat Products in Your Diet

On average, human breast milk calorie content is 56% fat, 39% carbohydrates, and 5% protein.

Carnivore milk is very different. Cheetah's, lion's and cat's milk, for example, have a calorie content of 51% fat, 14% carbohydrates, and 35% protein. [274]

If human milk is so low in protein, this would mean that although protein is necessary for human health, consuming high levels of protein by dietary means could have a hefty price on our health. See Chapter 3 for more detailed information on why excess protein is actually harmful to human health under the subheading "Was Meat the Magical Food That Allowed Humans to Succeed as a Species?"

In the modern world, we see high dietary consumption of animal protein, perhaps more than during any other time in human history, and it has been shown to have negative effects on human health as well as on the health of our planet. Through the domestication of animals, humans have been able to consume meat on a regular basis. But has this way of life proved to be good for us?

Is Red Meat Consumption At the Heart of Increased Rates of Modern Day Diseases?

Recent reports show that red meat consumption may be at the center of increased rates of heart disease as well as certain types of cancer.

In the history before agriculture we do not see much cardiovascular disease, and when examining gorillas and other apes, there is almost no evidence of heart disease in the wild. It is when these animals are put in zoos and fed modern Western diets rich in simple carbohydrates that they start to develop the whole array of what are known as modern day human diseases. [275, 277]

Fossil evidence shows us that high-status Egyptian Pharaohs had heart disease. Egyptian mummies, dating around 3500 years ago, were studied and nine of the sixteen mummies had evidence of having heart disease. In fact, the richer they were, the more buildup

Chapter 6 - The Theory Behind Reducing Meat Products in Your Diet

of fatty plaque and cholesterol they had in and on the artery walls (atherosclerosis). (276)

The pharaoh's diet was composed of a lot of fatty meats from cattle, ducks, and geese. They also used a lot of salt for food preservation and as a flavoring to their foods. Salt was very expensive at the time and considered a luxury.

In 1985, Dr. Caldwell B. Esselstyn Jr., began studying cholesterol levels and coronary disease on his patients. All of his patients participating in his study had severe, progressive, triple-vessel coronary heart disease as documented by angiography imaging techniques of blood vessels before entering the study. All participants were non-diabetic, non-hypertensive, and non-smokers. They ranged in age from 43 to 67 years. All participants were asked to adhere to a diet that derived less than 10% of its calories from fat. They were to avoid all oils, meat, fish, fowl, and dairy products, except for skim milk and nonfat yogurt. Their diet consisted mainly of grains, legumes, lentils, vegetables, and fruit. Participants were also encouraged to moderate their consumption of alcohol and caffeine. There were no prescribed exercise requirements. Among the eleven patients remaining in the ten year trial, six continued the diet and had no further coronary events, whereas the dropouts from the study who resumed their pre-study diet reported to have ten coronary events! (278)

But what about cancer? Does a reduction in animal protein also reduce the risk for cancer in humans?

My Own Personal Story with Meat Consumption

In fact, from my own personal experience, I am proof that eating a high meat diet made me more susceptible to cancer. I had been a vegetarian for many years and also a vegan at times, however, at one point in my life after coming across the Law Of Attraction in the movie *The Secret*, I thought to myself that perhaps nutrition was all in my mind, and presumed that if I ate as I wished but believed I would be healthy, then I would be healthy.

Chapter 6 - The Theory Behind Reducing Meat Products in Your Diet

Boy was I in for a surprise! I changed my eating patterns completely around during a period of four years I followed the common Western world diet. I stopped thinking about cruelty to animals, I stopped eating whole foods, and I began to conform to society. I did not realize the impact my decision would have on the world around me as well as on my own personal health. I ate hamburgers, white bread, white rice, and white pasta. I ate whipped cream, cheesecakes, and all the rest. I believe there is no need for any more details here as you get the picture. I thought that if everyone was eating these foods at the time, then maybe I was the crazy person for not consuming them.

After two and a half years on the average Western world diet came my first surprise in the form of uterine cancer.

I still did not see the connection with my diet until a second surprise showed up after four years into the average Western world diet in the form of thyroid cancer. I was operated on twice to remove the cancers, but after the second bout of cancer, I started searching for answers. I was amazed to learn that my diet was probably the culprit which had made me more susceptible to this disease. It was at this time that I devoted my spare time to researching the ideal diet for human consumption that will support health and longevity as well as a fit physique which I have happily gained in the process. No more need for dieting for me because by following **The Guerrilla Diet and Lifestyle Program**, I have, without any added effort on my part, reached my perfect weight. I have plenty of energy to fuel my life. This diet has truly changed my own personal life.

In fact, many publications, including research conducted by Dr. John McDougall, Dr. Dean Ornish, Dr. Alan Goldhamer, Dr. Neal Barnard, and many more, have shown a direct link between animal protein consumption and all of the Western world diseases including heart disease, diabetes, and cancers, but it is so hard for people to accept since most people have learned to love eating meat and presume that we are dependent on meat for our health.

Chapter 6 - The Theory Behind Reducing Meat Products in Your Diet

What Is It About Meat That We Love So Much?

Studies show that meat is quite tasteless and can even be bitter when eaten raw with no salt or sauces to complement its flavor. Cooking raw meat enhances the flavor of the meat by softening muscle fiber and weakening connective tissues to make it more palatable, but it still cannot be the reason behind our love for meat products.

Could we perhaps love eating meat because of its fat content?

I think that this *is* the reason. From an evolutionary prospective we crave fat because it is an excellent store of energy when food sources are low. Fat supplies the most calories per gram of food and this can really save us in times when food is sparse. 1 gram of fat = 9 calories of energy, unlike protein which supplies 3.8 calories per gram, and carbohydrates which supply 4 calories per gram. Humans instinctively crave fat due to millions of years of our history as hunter-gatherers and dealing with food scarcity. We humans have very efficient mechanisms that store fat in our bodies for the lean periods, and this is also the reason why it is so difficult to lose fat once it is gained.

The special thing about fat is that when food is scarce, the body can break down fatty deposits and release glucose to feed the brain ensuring our brains survival.

Meat from wild animals is very lean and low in fat, but nowadays meat from domesticated animals is rich in fat. The fatty deposits among muscle fibers soften the cooked meat and improve its flavor. Raw meat that is not spiced and uncooked is very difficult for a person to consume because the smell of the dead animal is so strong. Actually, carnivores salivate when they smell the strong scent of a dead animal; humans do not. But by cooking the meat, this smell disappears and the smell of fat excites our taste buds.

Today the food industry knows all too well about the natural human craving for fat. Farmers have begun genetically selecting animals that have a tendency to grow obese for domestication so that

Chapter 6 - The Theory Behind Reducing Meat Products in Your Diet

the huge companies and supermarkets will buy them. Farmers in this day and age have no choice but to comply with supermarket standards. They can only sell their foods to the supermarkets in modern countries because few others will buy them, and this leads to the big supermarkets dictating the future of farming.

Due to modern breeding methods to comply with supermarket standards, chickens, for example, suffer greatly. They are grown faster using growth hormones, and they reach their full adult size and weight in as little as five weeks, whereas in nature they grow to the same size in only twelve weeks. This escalated growth has many problems bound with it. Chicken bone development has not met the pace of this quick growth development. Their bones have less minerals, especially less calcium and phosphorus, thus making their bones brittle, causing them pain and great difficulty holding their weight and walking to get to the food and water they need to live. Some die from malnutrition or from simply being trampled upon by hardier chickens. Chicken meat now being sold is quite tasteless and nutrient-poor, but this is irrelevant to the seller who is looking to make the biggest profit from the faster growing birds.

Furthermore, the fat in chicken has increased to 17% of the total weight of the chicken whereas previously it was only around 6% of the weight in a natural chicken. People believe that by eating chicken meat they are eating a low fat alternative to red meat, when in fact, today's domesticated chickens are high in fat when they are bred and plumped through the modern system. Chickens are fed a high energy diet and raised in crowded living conditions, something very different from chickens living in their natural habitat. They are not given the option to roam the land freely so they do not exercise, their bones do not develop properly, and they do not burn off any fat. They become obese from these sedentary lifestyle and dietary habits, just as we humans do.

The meat consumed today is certainly not the natural wild meats consumed by early humans 200,000 years ago, even after cooking was introduced.

Moreover, even the fat composition of domesticated meat has changed over time. Previously animal fat was composed of both

Chapter 6 - The Theory Behind Reducing Meat Products in Your Diet

omega-3 and omega-6 fatty acids in equal proportions. Nowadays animal fat is especially rich in omega-6 fatty acids and very low in omega-3 fatty acids (considered beneficial in the prevention of heart disease) because of the intensive rearing methods commonly used by producers. [279, 280] Even as little as 100 years ago, the levels of omega-3 in meats were 170 mg/100 g of meat. Now they are only 20 mg/100 g of meat. *This shift in balance between omega-3 and omega-6 is thought to be the cause of many modern day ailments including the rise in mental health disorders.* [281] These include eating disorders, [282, 283, 284] which are a daily struggle for 10 million females and 1 million males in the US. Anorexia is the third most common chronic illness among adolescents. [285]

As hunter-gatherers, early humans chose foods by what they learned from their parents and what they were guided to eat by instinct. But over time most of us have lost this guidance instinct and so have our parents. Processed foods have made our taste buds less sensitive to the delicate taste of foods raised in nature. Our taste buds have become over stimulated from processed foods which are rich in fat, sugar, and salt, that gradually leads to their atrophy. Our taste buds have become accustomed to strong tasting foods rich in salt and flavorings which started when processed foods were introduced. Because processed foods are not natural and have gone through some form of processing treatment making them hardier with a longer shelf life, they are also less nutritious and have very little taste to them. As a solution to this problem, a new industry opened its doors, namely the food flavoring industry, which creates the flavor of foods and tricks our taste buds and made us more accustomed to stronger, unnatural flavors. [286]

So even if the taste of meat is very appealing, it becomes a question of whether the actual meat is the one that is appealing or if it is the flavoring added to it that makes it tasty. It is really amazing how even vegetarian or vegan processed foods can have the same taste as real meat due to the unnatural flavoring industry.

Chapter 6 - The Theory Behind Reducing Meat Products in Your Diet

Is Meat Consumption Beneficial to Our Health?

Now we understand that the excess in "high-quality" protein is not what we need for our health, and that our craving for fat is an evolutionary selection that is not useful for us in this day and age of plentitude. We also understand that the meat itself is not what we really love, but rather the flavorings added to it that make us love its flavor and its high fat content. Therefore it is time to look objectively at whether the consumption of high levels of meat is really beneficial to our health.

There is much evidence that shows that a high consumption of meat in the diet is detrimental to our health and to the health of our planet. As I have previously mentioned, throughout human evolution there was no other time when humans were consuming so much animal protein as now.

Meat Consumption and Infectious Diseases: The Facts

The world's deadliest infectious diseases nowadays are acute respiratory infections causing an estimated 4.3 million deaths a year. Diarrhea accounts for 1 in 9 child deaths worldwide, making it the second leading cause of death among children under the age of 5. [287] Tuberculosis accounted for around 1.5 million tuberculosis related deaths worldwide in 2013. [288]

These infectious diseases are largely transmitted by animals and animal products. The reason for this is that animals are being treated regularly, as a preventative measure, with antibiotics. Once people consume meat from animals that have been fed with antibiotics, resistance to these antibiotics is formed and antibiotics cannot be used effectively to cure disease when they are really needed.

Unlike the meat that earlier generations used to consume, most meat eaten today is different. In fact, the legal limit of real meat in "economy ground beef" is only 47%. [289]

Chapter 6 - The Theory Behind Reducing Meat Products in Your Diet

The way animals are reared now through domestication helps feed the billions of people on this planet to a surplus, but we are paying a hefty price for this sustenance.

The crowded living conditions of animals not only means that they are less fit and carry more fat, but it also means that diseases run rampant throughout the herds. Their litter where they spend their days and nights becomes full with urine and feces which is rich with ammonia. Ammonia burns their skin leading to ulcerations of the skin [290] which is very painful to them since they have pain receptors in the skin, just as humans do. This pain increases their stress hormone levels. Cramped living conditions also increase animal stress levels also leading to an increase in stress hormones in these animals. All of these conditions lead to a weakened immune system making these animals more prone to develop septicemia, (blood poisoning), caused by bacteria or their toxins, which can eventually be passed on to the person consuming these foods. The number of people developing septicemia in the Western world is significantly increasing with each passing year. [291] In the US, severe sepsis strikes more than one million Americans a year. [292] More people die from sepsis a year then from prostate cancer, breast cancer, and AIDS combined!

The crowded living conditions of domesticated animals have forced farmers to increase the use of antibiotics dramatically throughout the last few years to try and lower the infection rates between animals. Farmers began supplying these drugs to animals through their feed.

Most meat today is also pumped full of hormones which are used to make the animals grow faster. Although such drugs have all been individually tested and approved by the Food and Drug Administration (FDA) for animal use, the effects of these drugs on human health has not been investigated in sufficient length. Just to be "*on the safe side,*" farmers stop giving the drugs to animals several days before they are sent to be slaughtered, so that residues of these medications do not remain in the animals at high levels. But drug remains do persist and these drugs have been found in most supermarket meats when tested in a laboratory, even though they

Chapter 6 - The Theory Behind Reducing Meat Products in Your Diet

were within government acceptable limits. [293] Individual chemicals, hormones, or antibiotics may be within government limits separately, however, no one has tested what type of effect a combination of several chemicals, hormones, and antibiotics ingested from multiple animal products we eat has on our health. Instead, the toxicity of each drug is only tested separately.

The crowded living conditions of animals have monetary benefits for the farmer because the less space animals have, the less energy they use on movement and the less food they require, saving money for the farmers while providing more profit per animal sold. Also, the less energy the animals expend, the more tender their meat is because it is very fatty. In some places they are kept in such crowded conditions that the animals cannot even sit down, so they stand their entire life, only to be slaughtered at the end.

Eric Schlosser in his book/movie, *Fast Food Nation: The Dark Side of the All-American Meal* explains how the top four meat packing industries control 85% of the beef that's sold in the US. This industry is very powerful. He explains that there are thirteen meat slaughter houses that supply *all* of the meat that Americans consume in the US. His investigation showed that in a typical fast food hamburger you can find pieces of hundreds of different cattle because of the huge meat grinders that grind the meat from thousands of animals together. This also raises the risk of meat contamination. Sometimes meat may have fecal contamination leading to an increased risk of severe food poisoning. Bouts of food poisoning can have lifelong effects on human health. [294] The risk of meat containing contaminants depends largely on the number of cows making up the ground beef in the beef grinders. The greater the number of cows in the meat, the greater the chance of contracting something that shouldn't be in the meat in the first place.

Mad cow disease is an example of how a disease from animals can enter the food chain and affect the health of the human population. Mad cow disease was discovered in the United Kingdom in 1986 when it became a full-scale epidemic. The disease is caused by an infectious agent not destroyed even if the beef is cooked or heated. This infection causes deterioration of the brain tissue. [295]

Chapter 6 - The Theory Behind Reducing Meat Products in Your Diet

Mad cow disease is easily transmitted to human beings who ate beef contaminated with infected brain, spinal cord, digestive tract, or blood. [296, 297] In humans, there is mounting evidence that it may cause a variant illness called Creutzfeldt-Jakob Disease, which is not only fatal, but kills a person within fourteen months of diagnosis, By October 2009, 227 people had died from this disease worldwide. [298] Between 460,000 and 482,000 mad cow-infected animals had entered the human food chain before controls were introduced in 1989. [299] Encephalitis is also transferred from pigs to humans whom consume infected meat slices.

But there are other risks to our health from eating meat.

Meat Consumption and Cardiovascular Disease: The Facts

Red meat has high amounts of saturated fat and cholesterol. However, new research by Dr. Stanley Hazen and his team of scientists also shows that carnitine, found in the animal meat, when consumed in excess, gives rise to an artery-clogging compound called trimethylamine-N-oxide, or TMAO. Dr. Hazen says: "TMAO changes our cholesterol metabolism and contributes to the accumulation of cholesterol within the artery wall." In the research study they examined data from about 2,600 patients undergoing heart evaluations, and the link was clear. They found association between carnitine and risk for heart attack, stroke, and death." [302]

TMAO levels differed depending on the patient's diets. Researchers examined the blood TMAO levels of vegans, vegetarians, and meat-eaters after they ingested a uniform amount of carnitine, whether through a sirloin steak or vegan-friendly supplement. While meat-eaters made significant amounts of TMAO, vegans and vegetarians generated virtually none. Carnitine is used by some intestinal bacteria as food, and as Dr. Hazen says, "Vegans didn't have the microbes in their intestines to digest it." [302]

To confirm these results, they gave the meat eaters a week-long round of antibiotics to suppress the bacteria. When they re-administered carnitine, no one produced any TMAO, but after

Chapter 6 - The Theory Behind Reducing Meat Products in Your Diet

quitting antibiotics for a month, the meat eater's guts had repopulated with TMAO. "It was proof that gut microbes played a role in the metabolism of carnitine to produce this artery-clogging compound," Dr. Hazen says. When carnitine from our diet (or from supplementation) come into contact with certain bacteria in our intestines, they are metabolized into TMA, which makes its way to the liver through the portal circulation, where flavin-containing monooxygenases enzymes (FMOs) convert TMA into the unwanted TMAO. TMAO enters the bloodstream, where it participates in changes to cholesterol metabolism, vascular inflammation, and formation of unstable plaques in the arterial walls contributing to atherosclerosis, chronic kidney disease, and heart failure. Dr. Stanley Hazen and his team found a clear link between higher TMAO levels and elevated three-year risk of heart attack, stroke, and death.

Antibiotics aren't an effective treatment for heart disease. Dr. Hazen says: "You can't pop some pills with your steak to cancel out the carnitine since microbes develop antibiotic resistance quickly. But it is possible to shift your intestinal flora in the heart-healthy direction in just one or two months by adopting a vegetarian or vegan diet". [300]

Another study followed 37,698 men from the Health Professionals Follow-up Study in the US (1986-2008) and 83,644 women from the Nurse's Health Study in the US (1980-2008), who were at baseline free of cardiovascular disease and cancer. Diet was assessed by validated food-frequency questionnaires and updated every four years.

They concluded that red meat consumption was associated with an increased risk of total cardiovascular disease and cancer mortality. Substitution of other healthy protein sources for red meat was associated with a lower mortality risk. [301]

Another study comparing analysis of 5 prospective studies, with data from 76,172 men and women, examined the death rates from common diseases of vegetarians with those of non-vegetarians with similar lifestyles. In these studies, 27,808 vegetarians, who did not eat any meat or fish were included. Death rate ratios at ages 16-89 years were calculated and all results were adjusted for age, sex,

Chapter 6 - The Theory Behind Reducing Meat Products in Your Diet

and smoking status. There were, all together, 8,330 deaths after a mean of 10.6 years of follow-up. They found that mortality from heart disease was 24% lower in vegetarians than in non-vegetarians, and that the lower mortality from heart disease among vegetarians was greater at younger ages and was restricted to those who had followed their current diet for over five years. [302]

Meat Consumption and Diabetes: The Facts

Recent statistics combining results from different studies have identified positive associations between red meat consumption and an elevated risk of Type 2 diabetes mellitus. [303, 304]

A recent report by Professor of Epidemiology, Frank Hu, and Dr. An Pan, a research fellow from the Harvard School of Public Health, published a paper in 2013 in the Journal of the American Medical Association (JAMA) in Internal Medicine showing evidence that eating red or processed meat can, over time, increase the risk of developing Type 2 diabetes. Dr. Pan writes: "Specifically, 3.5 ounces of red meat (the equivalent to one hot dog), or 1.8 ounces of processed meat (the equivalent to 2 slices of bacon) daily, led to a 19% and 51% increase in diabetes risk, respectively." [305] They found that just by increasing red meat intake by three extra servings every week there was an associated elevated risk of Type 2 diabetes mellitus by 48% compared with the reference group that had no change in red meat intake. By reducing red meat consumption by three servings per week they found 14% lower risk of Type 2 diabetes mellitus. Their evidence concluded that increasing red meat consumption over time is associated with an elevated subsequent risk of Type 2 diabetes mellitus, and the association was shown to be partly mediated by body weight. By limiting red meat consumption over time you will find benefits for Type 2 diabetes mellitus prevention. [305]

Chapter 6 - The Theory Behind Reducing Meat Products in Your Diet

In another study, researchers looked at long-term health data of twenty years of follow-up from three Harvard University cohorts that included:

1. Over 26,300 men participating in one Health Professionals Follow-Up Study.
2. More than 48,700 women in a Nurses Health Study.
3. Slightly over 74,000 women from a different Nurses Health Study.

During that time, 7,540 people developed Type 2 diabetes. Within each cohort, those who ate more red meat as the study progressed showed higher rates of diabetes than those whose consumption didn't change.

Those who added more than half a serving of red meat per day from the time the study started showed a 48% greater risk of Type 2 diabetes at the next four-year checkup compared with participants who did not increase intake during that time. On the other hand, people who lowered their red meat consumption by more half a serving each day from the start of the study, enjoyed a 14% lower risk of having Type 2 diabetes over the course of the entire study compared with those who didn't change how much red meat they ate. Rates of diabetes were higher among people who consumed mostly processed meats such as salami and hot dogs compared with those who ate unprocessed red meat. [306]

Professor Frank Hu says that even though it is "...difficult to pinpoint one compound or ingredient..." linking meat with diabetes risk, three components of red meat including sodium, nitrites, and iron, are probably involved. Sodium is well known to increase blood pressure, but it also causes insulin resistance. Nitrites and nitrates have also been shown to increase insulin resistance and to impair the function of the pancreatic beta-cells that produce insulin. Iron, although an essential mineral, can cause pancreatic beta-cell damage in individuals with hereditary hemochromatosis (a disorder in which the gastrointestinal tract absorbs too much iron). Heme iron, the readily absorbable type found in meat at high levels, can lead to oxidative stress and cellular damage, as well as systemic, chronic inflammation in some people.

Chapter 6 - The Theory Behind Reducing Meat Products in Your Diet

Meat Consumption and Cognitive Function: The Facts

Alzheimer's disease is a generalized degeneration of the brain that leads to progressive mental deterioration occurring in middle or old age. It is the most common cause of premature senility. Most researchers believe the disease is caused by a disruption of signaling between neurons (a type of brain cell) or a destruction of them as we age.

A study by Dr. George Bartzokis, a professor of psychiatry at the Semel Institute for Neuroscience and Human Behavior at UCLA, suggests a third possible cause: iron accumulation.

Dr. Bartzokis and his colleagues looked at two areas of the brain in patients with Alzheimer's. They compared the hippocampus, which is known to be damaged during the early stages of Alzheimer's disease, and the thalamus, an area that is generally not affected until the later stages of the disease. Using brain-imaging techniques, they found that iron is increased in the hippocampus and is associated with tissue damage in that area, but they did not observe increased iron in the thalamus. [307]

Meat contains a lot of iron. Although iron is essential for cell function, too much of it can promote oxidative damage to which the brain is especially vulnerable. When red meat is eaten in excess, it may raise levels of iron in the brain and may increase the risk of developing Alzheimer's disease. When iron accumulates in the brain, myelin, the fatty tissue that coats nerve fibers, is destroyed. This disrupts brain cell communication and signs of Alzheimer's disease begin to appear. [308]

Meat Consumption and Cancer: The Facts

Quite a few studies have provided evidence of red meat potentially causing cancer. Although the results vary, studies from around the world have clearly suggested that a high consumption of meat is directly linked to an increased risk of one specific cancer, namely colon cancer.

Chapter 6 - The Theory Behind Reducing Meat Products in Your Diet

Evidence comes from two large 2005 studies: one from Europe [618], the other from the United States [619]. The European research group tracked 478,000 men and women who were free of cancer when the study began. The people who ate the most red meat (about 5 ounces a day or more = 1000 grams per week) were about a third more likely to develop colon cancer than those who ate the least red meat (less than an ounce a day on average = less than 200 grams per week). Their consumption of chicken did not influence risk one way or the other, but a high consumption of fish appeared to reduce the risk of colon cancer by about a third.

The US study added important information about the effects of long-term meat consumption. 148,610 people between the ages of fifty and seventy-four showed that a high consumption of red and processed meats substantially increased the risk of colorectal cancer.

Furthermore, a meta-analysis of twenty-nine studies of meat consumption and colon cancer concluded that a high consumption of red meat increases risk of colon cancer by 28%, and a high consumption of processed meat increases the risk by 20%. [611]
Humans are not made to consume meat in large quantities. But by what mechanisms does meat have the ability to cause cancer in humans?

Scientists from England offer an explanation. They recruited healthy volunteers who were placed on one of three diets for a period of fifteen to twenty-one days. The first diet contained about 14 ounces (400 grams) of red meat a day. The second diet was strictly vegetarian, and the third diet contained large amounts of both red meat and dietary fiber. The researchers found high levels of *N-nitroso compounds* (NOCs), which are carcinogens (potential cancer-causing chemicals), in the stool specimens of twenty-one volunteers who consumed the high-meat diet. The twelve volunteers who ate vegetarian food excreted low levels of NOCs, and the thirteen who ate meat and high-fiber diets produced intermediate amounts.

The researchers then retrieved cells from the lining of the colon shed into the stool. The cells from people eating the high-meat diet contained a large number of cells that had NOC-induced DNA damage; the stools of vegetarians had the lowest number of cells with

Chapter 6 - The Theory Behind Reducing Meat Products in Your Diet

damaged genetic material, and the people who ate high-meat, high-fiber diets produced intermediate numbers of damaged cells. [309] To summarize, *N-nitroso compounds* produced from meat-rich diets lead to genetic damage of cells, which causes unhealthy cancerous cells to appear in greater quantities than the body has the ability to control.

Furthermore, hormones now being added to red meat boost breast cancer risk according to a large study published in the Archives of Internal Medicine. Red meat intake and breast cancer risk were assessed among premenopausal women aged twenty-six to forty-six years in the Nurse's Health Study II. During twelve years of follow-up of over 90,000 premenopausal women, they found that the greater the red meat intake, the higher the risk of breast cancers that were estrogen and progesterone receptor positive. In comparison, those eating three or fewer servings per week of red meat were much less at risk. Women who ate more than 1.5 daily servings of red meat, including beef, pork, and lamb, were nearly twice as likely to be at risk than women who ate three or fewer servings per week. Researchers believe the hormones or hormone-like compounds in red meat increase cancer risk by attaching to specific hormone receptors on certain tumors. They conclude that a higher red meat intake may be a risk factor for breast cancer among premenopausal women. [310]

Dr.'s Farvid, Takemi, fellow and associate professor in the department of nutrition at the Harvard School of Public Health, in her research to investigate the association between dietary protein sources in early adulthood and risk of breast cancer in an analysis of nearly 88,800 women, concluded that heavy consumption of red meat was strongly associated with a relative risk for breast cancer (22% higher than that seen among women at the lowest end of the meat-eating spectrum). Dr. Takemi's study reveals that it is also the cooking of the meat that increases the risk for suffering from breast cancer. Dr. Takemi says that: "Carcinogenic by-products such as heterocyclic amines and polycyclic aromatic hydrocarbons, created during high temperatures cooking of meat; as well as animal fat and heme iron from red meat; and hormone residues of the externally provided growth hormones given to cattle are some of the mechanisms that may explain the positive association between high intake of red meat and risk of breast cancer." [311] Dr. Takemi concludes that by substituting one serving a day of legumes for one serving a day of red meat, there was a 15% lower risk of breast cancer among all women and a 19% lower risk among premenopausal women. [311]

Meat Consumption and the Environment: The Facts

Red meat impacts the environment more than any other food we eat, mainly because livestock require much more land, food, water, and energy in order to grow and be transported to awaiting customers than plants need.

Producing a four-ounce (quarter pound or 113 gram) hamburger, for example, requires:
- 7 pounds (3.2 kg) of grain or forage a day.
- 53 gallons (200 liters) of drinking water for the cows and irrigation water to feed the crops that feed the animals.
- 75 square feet (7 square meters) for grazing and growing the crops to feed the animals.
- 1,036 BTUs for feed production and transport. (The energy content of fuel is expressed in BTUs which are a measure of agricultural energy production, the amount of energy needed to cool or heat one pound of water by one degree Fahrenheit.) This is enough energy to power a microwave for eighteen minutes.

In order to raise animals, many forests are being burned down and cleared to make more land available. This is a very profitable decision for the land owner, but less so to the world at large. Deforestation increases global warming which in itself has had devastating effects on agriculture. It is much more difficult to grow crops in hotter conditions that arise due to global warming.

Both processed foods and high animal proteins are not only the worst foods for our health, they are absolutely harmful for our planet.

Chapter 6 - The Theory Behind Reducing Meat Products in Your Diet

By reducing the amount of meat and dairy foods consumed, and lowering the consumption of processed foods, we are reducing energy usage *and* land wastage in a major way. By reducing the amount of meat we consume, we are taking the first major step in claiming back our health and the health of planet earth as well as the livelihood of our neighbors on the planet, the animals.

Fish Consumption: The Facts

Fish consumption is considered to be a healthy alternative to eating meat. But is this really the case and do we need to consume fish to increase our omega-3 essential fatty acid intake?

Some fish available today are largely contaminated due to elevated levels of pesticides that run off into the bodies of water from agricultural land. There is also evidence linking fish contamination to cancer. [312, 313] In fact, many fish themselves are increasingly suffering from cancer. [314]

As I stated in Chapter 4 under the heading "*Gorilla and Human Omega-3 and Omega-6 Fatty Acid Requirements,*" the fatty acids omega-3 and omega-6 are essential to human health because the body cannot produce them; they must come from dietary sources. In the diet, omega-3 and omega-6 consumed should be at a healthy ratio of 1:1 as is found in the natural gorilla and ancient human diets. The modern Western world diet consists of a ratio of up to 1:20 of omega-3 to omega-6! Excess of each of these fatty acids will suppress the absorption or transformation of the other fatty acid. Excess of any of these fatty acids is also harmful to the body and causes many problems in the long term. Polyunsaturated fatty acids regulate inflammatory processes. Inflammation is critical because it stimulates the immune system during infections, viruses, or traumas. However, chronic inflammation is when the inflammatory process gets out of hand. We only need polyunsaturated fatty acids in small amounts to control some essential inflammatory pathways, but not in excess. Today, inflammation is at the source of almost every modern health problem. The fact that excess polyunsaturated fatty acid consumption promotes general and chronic inflammation is an important fact to remember.

So how can we control our intake of fatty acids to ensure we get them at the right levels for our health? And from what food sources?

As explained in Chapter 4, our body makes omega-3 and omega-6 from alpha-linolenic acid (ALA) found in nuts, seeds, potatoes, corn, and grains, and from linoleic acid (LA) found in plants sources like flax seeds, walnuts, chia seeds, kale, spinach, and other green leafy vegetables as well as beans. Once eaten, the body converts ALA first into eicosapentaenoic acid (EPA) and then into docosahexaenoic acid (DHA) an omega-3 fatty acid in a more usable form for the body. The body also converts LA to gamma linoleic acid (GLA), a more usable form of omega-6 fatty acid for the body. This process of conversion works in response to the body's fatty acid requirements and only a small fraction of the ALA ends up being transformed to a usable form of omega-3, DHA.

Although our bodies can get their fatty acid needs met directly with the usable form of omega-3 and omega-6 by eating foods higher up the food chain such as fish, wild meat, and eggs, are these really a better choice? When we consume lots of fish, meat, or eggs per week we are getting polyunsaturated fatty acids in excess and this leads to problems. For example, EPA determines the fluidity of our blood, and in excess it leads to thrombosis and stroke. When we receive the ready-made omega-3 and omega-6 we cannot control the amount of polyunsaturated fatty acids that we have in our body. When we are getting our fatty acid intake from leafy green vegetables, nuts, and seed sources, our body will produce only the amount of polyunsaturated fatty acids that we really need and no more.

Omega-3 polyunsaturated fatty acid intake from walnuts, flax seeds, chia seeds, and green leafy vegetable is very important for our health. Excess omega-6 in the diet through high consumption of meat, eggs, and farmed fish may suppress the absorption or transformation of omega-3 fatty acids. Omega-3 polyunsaturated fatty acids exert an anti-inflammatory action by promoting the resolution of the inflammatory cycle. Omega-3 fatty acids also play a role in normal brain development and function. [315] Omega-3 polyunsaturated fatty acids help in preventing heart disease. [316, 317] DHA and EPA have also been proven beneficial for Alzheimer's disease, [318] Parkinson's disease [319, 320] stroke, [321] and psoriasis. [322] Therefore it is important to get the fatty acids in correct proportions, and not in excess by consuming them through vegetarian sources and allowing our bodies to produce only the required amounts of usable omega-3 and omega-6 fatty acids rather than coping with excessive amounts.

Meat Consumption and Animal Welfare: The Facts

One more thing important to consider when we are consuming meat products is the welfare of our neighbor's on this planet, the animals.

Sometimes we easily forget that the steak, fish, or chicken on our plate was part of a living creature. The path that animals go through from birth until they become a serving at dinnertime is filled with unbelievable cruelty that I will not detail here. Paul Shapiro, the vice-president of Farm Animal Protection at the Humane Society of the United States (HSUS), says that "Many standard agribusiness practices are so inhumane, so out of step with mainstream American values about how animals should be treated, they would be illegal if the victims were dogs or cats." Recent HSUS undercover investigations have revealed appalling abuses of cattle, pigs, chickens, and turkeys. Paul Shapiro says that sadly, these cruelties are common in factory farms across the nation.

He continues by pointing out that each of us can stand up for these animals every time we sit down to eat. By making better food choices, we all have the power to create a more humane society. [323]

It is not easy to change any habit, especially to habits that are different from the ones we grew up with and have been passed down from generation to generation in our families. At first, we may go through a period of severe discomfort, but know that every step you make in the right direction is to be praised and makes a difference. Remember, there is no need to give up meat entirely unless this is your choice. (***The Guerrilla Diet and Lifestyle Program*** recommendations for animal products are covered in Section 2 of this book.)

It doesn't matter if your reasons for reducing animal products from your diet come from your concern for your own health, concern over the welfare of animals, or from concern for our planet. You should know that you are making a major difference to all of these fields once you make the decision to reduce meat products from your menu. Then you can safely take pride in your commitment to the betterment of all.

Chapter 7

The Theory Behind Removing Milk Products From Your Diet

"No one asks the cow or the chicken where it gets its protein."

— John Salley

Milk is a prime source of two very important nutrients: calcium and potassium.

Calcium is one of the most important minerals for the human body as it helps form and maintain healthy teeth and bones. Ninety-nine percent of the calcium in the human body is stored in the teeth and bones where it provides hardness for tissue strength. The remaining 1% is found in the blood and other tissues [324] where it assists in numerous other functions including blood clotting, muscle contraction, vasodilatation, hormonal secretion, the transmission of nerve impulses, as an essential intracellular messenger, and playing key roles in cell signalling and maintaining a normal heart rhythm. [325, 326]

The weakening of bones due to low levels of calcium and potassium leads to osteoporosis. Each year osteoporosis causes more than 1.5 million human bone fractures, including 300,000 broken hips in Americans 65 years or older of which 20-30% will die within 12 months. On the other hand there is growing evidence that consuming a lot of milk and other dairy products has little effect on bone density and may, in fact, contribute to osteoporosis and other health problems including heart disease, cancer, and more. Let's look at the facts.

Lactose Intolerance: The Facts

The origins of milking dates back only 7000 years. [327]

Cow's milk is not an ideal food for humans for a number of reasons.

In order to digest the sugar found in dairy products called lactose, humans need an enzyme that helps break down lactose into usable components for our body. This enzyme is called Lactase and is located in the small intestine where it is responsible for digestion of the sugar lactose. Lactase activity is high and vital during infancy, but in most mammals, including most humans, lactase activity declines after the weaning phase making the person unable to breakdown lactose to its usable components, thereby rendering the person intolerant to lactose.

Professor Ron Pinhasi and his colleagues from the University College Dublin Earth Institute and School of Archaeology, examined DNA from ancient fossil remains in search of known genetic markers including lactose intolerance. Their findings show that ancient Europeans remained intolerant to lactose for 5,000 years after they adopted animal domestication practices for milk and 4,000 years after the onset of cheese-making among Central European Neolithic farmers. [328]

Ancient Europeans domesticated animals such as cows, sheep, and goats without having yet developed the genetic tolerance for drinking milk from mammals. [329, 330]

So why did people begin dairy farming if they could not utilize milk properly as a food source 7000 years ago?

Researchers suggest that ancient Europeans may have practiced dairying not to drink milk, but to consume milk products such as cheese and yogurt which have considerably less lactose. [331]

Chapter 7 - The Theory Behind Removing Milk Products From Your Diet

Cheese production evolved quickly after the development of dairy farming. The first direct signs of cheese making were found in broken pieces of ancient ceramic material from Poland by Peter Bogucki, an archaeologist at Princeton University in the 1980s. He and his collaborator, Mélanie Salque, a chemist at the University of Bristol, UK, found fragments of pottery with small holes in them and realized these were used as sieves to strain the curds from milk. He recalls: "There weren't many of them, but there were a few at just about every site." He reasoned that Neolithic farmers had found a way to use their herds for more than milk or meat, and had started to make cheese which is much lower in lactose. [332, 327, 333, 334]

The processes that make cheese and yogurt also help break down lactose in the milk.

Most of the current world population remains lactose intolerant, unable as adults to digest the complex milk sugar lactose found in cow's milk and dairy products, leading to side effects such as diarrhea, cramping, bloating, and gas. However, while cheese is a dairy product, it is relatively low in lactose, which helped people take advantage of animal milk, a food one could sustainably secure even in extreme and rapidly changing weather conditions of northern Europe.

The presence of dairying over many generations helped set the stage for an evolutionary change in certain populations, like northern Europeans, making them lactase persistent, meaning that the enzyme lactase, which breaks down lactose, remains active well into adulthood, enabling them to digest lactose also as adults. [335] This genetic change is probably due to natural selection of the fittest because when food supply was sparse, the ability to continue to tolerate lactose helped people in the cold European continent to have a sustainable food source by milking cows and making cheeses.

However, early dairy farming was expensive and time consuming. Bulls were needed to get the cow pregnant, and the gestation period for a cow is about nine months long. Cows gave birth and then their milk was used to feed their young calves as well as the people who raised the cattle. Cows also typically have only one baby at a time and milk production lasts around four years. But when the weather was not stable enough to permit regular growth of many other food sources, northern Europeans relied on cows and goats for milk. It is mostly in these populations that we still see the people with lactose persistence. However, in most populations throughout the world, lactose intolerance is still prevalent in humans.

Table 4: Lactose Intolerant Statistics Today

Total percentage of adults who have a decreased lactase activity in adulthood	75%
Total number of Americans who are lactose intolerant	40 million
Total percent of all African-American, Jewish, Mexican-American, and Native American Adults who are lactose intolerant	75%
Total percent of Asian-Americans that are lactose intolerant	90%
Average amount of time it takes for side effects of lactose intolerance to occur after intake	30 min.

As we can see from the table above, most humans remain unable to digest lactose after childhood. For them, eating or drinking dairy products causes the above mentioned problems. Ninety percent of Asians, seventy-five percent of Africans and Native Americans, and fifty percent of Hispanics are lactose intolerant, compared to only about fifteen percent of people from Northern European descent. The number of lactose intolerant people in the world will grow in this coming century with the main population growth expected in Africa and Asia in comparison with the European population.

But, as we can see, there are people that *can* tolerate lactose, so why should such people refrain from consuming milk products when they are such an important calcium source?

Chapter 7 - The Theory Behind Removing Milk Products From Your Diet

Where Can People Get Their Calcium Requirements If Not from Milk and Dairy Products?

The body can receive its calcium requirements by consuming calcium rich foods including dark leafy greens, seeds, dried beans, or drinking water, which all have varying amounts of absorbable calcium. Calcium is found at high levels in dairy foods, however, this calcium is not well absorbed by the body. For the body to absorb calcium efficiently there has to be a relatively equal amount of magnesium present in the food source. Milk only contains a small amount of magnesium, so the body cannot make use of all of the calcium contained within it. In reality, only about 25% of dairy calcium from milk can be absorbed. The remaining 75% can end up causing problems in the body leading to kidney stones, plaque build-up in the arteries, gout, and can be a contributing factor for arthritis. Calcium found in dark leafy vegetables including broccoli, brussel sprouts, kale, turnip greens, mustard greens, spinach, chicory, collard greens, dandelion greens, Swiss chard, and arugula are more absorbable than calcium from dairy products.

If there is not enough calcium in our diet and blood levels of calcium drop too low, the body will then get its required calcium by pulling it out from bones. (Please go to the chart: *Foods Rich in Calcium Recommended by **The Guerrilla Diet and Lifestyle Program*** in Chapter 9 for a detailed list of plant based foods rich in calcium and magnesium.)

Bone is living tissue which is always in flux. Human bones are constantly being broken down and being built up in a process known as remodeling. Bone cells called osteoblasts build bone, while other bone cells called osteoclasts break down bone. In healthy individuals who get enough calcium and physical activity, bone production exceeds bone destruction up to around the age of thirty. After that, destruction typically exceeds production. [336]

Dairy Foods and Osteoporosis: The Facts

Osteoporosis is the weakening of bones caused by a drastic imbalance between levels of bone creation and bone destruction. People typically lose bone tissue as they age, despite consuming the recommended intake of calcium necessary to maintain optimal bone health. In fact, receiving higher amounts of calcium over a long period of time raises the risk of kidney stones in some people, one of the most common disorders of the urinary tract today, [337] and excess calcium has not been proven to reduce osteoporosis. But why?

Achieving adequate calcium intake and maximizing bone stores through impact exercising during the time when bone is rapidly deposited (up to age thirty) provides an important foundation for the future, but it will not prevent bone loss later in life. The loss of bone with ageing is the result of several factors including genetic and dietary factors, physical activity levels, and levels of circulating hormones (estrogen in women and testosterone in men).

Maximum calcium retention studies, which examine the maximum amount of calcium that can be forced into bones, suggest a daily high calcium requirement. To ensure that 95% of the population gets this much calcium, the National Academy of Sciences established very high calcium recommended intake levels:

- 1,000 milligrams/day for those aged nineteen to fifty.
- 1,200 milligrams/day for those aged fifty or over.
- 1,000 milligrams/day for pregnant or lactating adult women.

But the maximum calcium retention studies are short term studies and therefore have major limitations.

The results from long-term studies show an entirely different picture. While they do not question the importance of calcium in maximizing bone strength, these studies suggest that high calcium intake doesn't actually appear to lower a person's risk for osteoporosis.

For example, in the two large ongoing Harvard studies of male health professionals and female nurses which I mentioned in the previous chapter, individuals who drank one glass of milk or less per week were at no greater risk of breaking a hip or forearm than

Chapter 7 - The Theory Behind Removing Milk Products From Your Diet

were those who drank two or more glasses per week. [338, 339] When researchers combined the data from the Harvard studies with other large prospective studies, they still found no association between calcium intake from dairy products and fracture risk. [340] A recent study showed that higher milk consumption during teenage years was not associated with a lower risk of hip fracture in older adults. [341] A 2005 review published in *Pediatrics* magazine showed that milk consumption does not improve bone integrity in children. [342] In a more recent study, researchers tracked the diets, physical activity, and stress fracture incidences of adolescent girls for seven years, and concluded that dairy products and calcium do not prevent stress fractures in adolescent girls. [343]

Additional evidence further supports the idea that American adults may not need as much calcium as is currently recommended. For example, in countries such as India, Japan, and Peru where average daily calcium intake is as low as 300 milligrams per day (less than a third of the US recommendation for adults aged nineteen to fifty), the incidence of bone fractures is quite low. Of course, these countries differ in other important bone-health factors as well, such as dietary intake of legumes, levels of physical activity and amount of sunlight which could also account for their low fracture rates. [344] Similarly, the Harvard Nurses' Health Study, which followed more than 72,000 women for 12 years, found no protective effect of increased milk consumption on fracture risk. [345]

Studies show that one of the leading causes of osteoporosis is consuming too much dietary animal protein in the form of dairy products. [346, 347, 348, 349, 350] Furthermore, the amount of calcium absorbed from foods can vary tremendously depending on total dietary calcium intake and the sources of dietary calcium.

Cows get their calcium from a high consumption of plant foods. Grass is rich in calcium. The calcium from plants is also rich in magnesium necessary for the body to absorb and utilize the calcium. The calcium in cow's milk is magnesium poor and the countries with the highest amount of milk/dairy consumption have been found to have the highest rates of osteoporosis. [345]

Chapter 7 - The Theory Behind Removing Milk Products From Your Diet

Also, the amount of calcium content in foods varies significantly in different parts of the globe and even between different foods grown in the same country in different habitats.

Both the nutrient variation in foods and the variation in nutrient absorption depending on the total diet of an individual, work together and intensify each other. Furthermore, interactions among individual nutrients in foods are also substantial and dynamic and must be considered.

A review of nutrient-nutrient interactions showed that excess calcium interferes with leukocyte function by displacing magnesium ions, thereby reducing immune function and cell adhesion. [351]

However, I believe that by focusing on specific nutrients found in milk, we are missing the bigger picture. Our bodies are a whole system with everything working together to make the body function in the best possible way. Foods are not just a collection of nutrients, but are complex and influence our health in many more ways than just the sum of their nutrients. The real question to be asked is whether dairy foods are really good for our health.

Milk and dairy products may not be the ideal food source they are thought to be!

Dairy Foods and IQ: The Facts

Of all mammals, human milk has the lowest ratio of casein to whey. Human milk has only 1.2 mg/liter protein content, 4.2% fat, 7.0% lactose, and supplies 72 kcal of energy per 100 grams. [352] The protein found in breast milk is mostly whey which is easier to digest than casein, the main protein found in cow's milk (80%). Cow's milk contains, on average, 3.4% protein, 3.6% fat, and 4.6% lactose, and supplies 66 kcal of energy per 100 grams.

The time required for a human baby to double its birth weight is 120 days. This is a very long period in comparison with a cow. A baby calf doubles its birth weight is just 47 days.

Chapter 7 - The Theory Behind Removing Milk Products From Your Diet

Rats have a very high protein content in their milk (11.8 mg/liter), and baby rats double their weight in only 4.5 days.

The protein content of milk allows the body to grow very fast. Human babies are helpless when they are born, unlike cows who can, within a number of minutes, begin to walk and find their food source. Human babies, on the other hand, need to first develop their brains and then increase their body weight to survive. Therefore the milk of a cow, which is intended to make the calf grow quickly to its large size, is less directed towards making the brain of the cow develop. Human milk is geared towards increasing brain development and less for musculoskeletal growth.

Brain tissue consists largely of fat which insulates nerve fibers in the form of myelin sheaths. Human breast milk contains cholesterol which is needed to make nerve tissue in the growing brain. The fats in breast milk are practically self-digesting, since breast milk also contains the enzyme lipase which breaks down the fat. Fat in human milk has large amounts of omega-3 fatty acids that are important for brain development. Omega-3 fatty acids are found in much higher concentrations in human milk than in cow's milk.

The levels of this fatty acid in breast milk depend on the mother's consumption of omega-3 rich foods. So important are these brain-building fats that if mother's diet doesn't provide enough of them through her diet for her milk, the breast tissue may produce them.

Breast milk is also higher in lactose compared to cow's milk. Lactose is broken down in the body into glucose and galactose, which is a valuable nutrient for brain tissue development. We know from animal studies that the more intelligent species of mammals have greater amounts of lactose in their milk. Soy-based and other lactose-free formulas obviously contain no lactose at all and are therefore less beneficial for human babies than mother breast milk.

The protein of human breast milk has high amounts of amino acid taurine which plays an important role in the development of brain tissue and eyes. This amino acid is low in cow's milk.

The breastfeeding process itself may also benefit a child's brain development because it varies more than the bottle-feeding experience. The taste changes, the texture changes, and it requires more energy to consume. Breastfeeding also takes longer and thus provides more closeness between the baby and mother. [353]

Children raised on cow's milk were found to have a lower IQ than children raised on mothers milk. [354] Cow milk is intended for cows and does not meet the nutrient requirements for human babies and may even lead to toxicity in infants.

In an editorial, Dimitri A. Christakis of the Seattle Children's Hospital Research Institute, stated that breastfeeding an infant for the first year of life would be expected to increase his or her IQ by about four points or one-third of a standard deviation. [355] Other observational studies report positive associations of breastfeeding with later intelligence. [356, 357, 358, 359]

The truth is that it is very unnatural for any animal to live off the milk of another animal. Milk from one mammal is made in the best way to provide the offspring of that animal the best nutrition. As we have seen in this chapter and in the table in Chapter 6, milk from different animals has very different compositions. The biochemical make-up of cow's milk is perfectly suited to turn a 65-pound newborn calf into a 400-pound cow in one year. It contains three times more protein and seven times more mineral content than human milk. On the other hand, human milk has ten times more essential fatty acids, three times the amount of selenium, twice as much taurine, and half the calcium of cow's milk.

Dairy Foods and Cardiovascular Disease: The Facts

Many dairy products are high in saturated fats, and a high saturated fat intake after infancy is a risk factor for cardiovascular disease. Dairy products contribute significant amounts of cholesterol and saturated fat to the diet. [360] Vegans and vegetarians have been proven to be healthier with regard to cardiovascular status than meat eaters. [361] But when comparing cholesterol and cardiovascular status between vegetarians and vegans, vegans have shown to have

Chapter 7 - The Theory Behind Removing Milk Products From Your Diet

better cardiovascular status than vegetarians who consume dairy products. [362]

While it's true that most dairy products are now available in fat-reduced or non-fat options, the saturated fat that is removed is usually replaced with sugar or chemical sweeteners to compensate for the lack of taste that comes from the removal of fats. Even though the fat is reduced in some dairy products, fat still forms a significant part of these foods.

So how much fat does milk really contain?
- In whole milk, 49% of the calories are from fat.
- In "2%" milk, 35% of the calories are from fat.
- In skim milk, 6% of the calories are from fat.
- In cheddar cheese, 74% of the calories are from fat.
- In butter, 100% of the calories are from fat.

Comparisons between a diet low in saturated fats with plenty of fresh fruit and vegetables, and the typical diet of someone living in the Western developed world, show that in the former there is a 73% reduction in the risk of new major cardiac events. [363]

The role of diet is crucial in the development and prevention of cardiovascular disease. Diet is one of the key things you can change that will impact all cardiovascular risk factors.

Dairy Foods and Iron Status: The Facts

Iron status is significantly impaired when whole cow's milk is introduced into the diet of young infants. [364] This is the period of greatest iron need and highest prevalence of iron deficiency anemia. [365] A study of 1311 children pointed that an increase in cow's milk consumption was associated with decreasing serum ferritin. [366] In fact, the research shows that babies who are fed on whole cow's milk showed an increase in intestinal blood loss of up to 30%. [364] What leads these infants to bleed after the consumption of cow milk? The high levels of protein in cow's milk are very difficult to digest. The protein casein found in cow's milk, unlike the whey protein found in human breast milk, irritates the gut wall and causes internal bleeding which leads to iron loss. The same also occurs in adults.

Dairy Foods and Infertility: The Facts

The World Health Organization (WHO), the American Society for Reproductive Medicine (ASRM), and the American College of Obstetricians and Gynecologists (ACOG) recognize infertility as a disease. Infertility is a disease that results in the abnormal functioning of the male or female reproductive system. Eleven point nine percent of American women receive infertility services during their lifetime, and one in eight couples (or 12% of married women) has trouble getting pregnant or sustaining a pregnancy. [367]

Dairy foods have been found to impair fertility by affecting ovulatory function. A study prospectively followed 18,555 married, premenopausal women without a history of infertility, who attempted a pregnancy or became pregnant during an eight year period. Their diet was assessed and the results showed that a high intake of low-fat dairy foods increase the risk of infertility. [368]

Dairy Foods and Cancer: The Facts

A recent pooled analysis of twelve prospective cohort studies, which included more than 500,000 adult women, found that women who had high intakes of lactose in adulthood, equivalent to three or more servings of milk per day, had a higher risk of ovarian cancer, compared to women with the lowest lactose intakes. [369] In a case-control study, consumption of dairy foods was linked to a highly significant trend for increasing ovarian cancer risk. They concluded that lactose consumption may be a dietary risk factor, especially when dairy consumption exceeds the levels of the enzyme beta galactosidase and its ability to break down galactose. The galactose levels build up in the blood and other tissues, including the ovaries. [370]

Moreover, some researchers have also hypothesized that modern industrial milk production practices have changed milk's hormone composition in ways that could increase the risk of hormone-related cancers. [371]

Chapter 7 - The Theory Behind Removing Milk Products From Your Diet

A diet high in calcium from dairy products has been implicated as a probable risk factor for prostate cancer and prostate infections. [372] In a Harvard study of male health professionals, men who drank two or more glasses of milk a day were almost twice as likely to develop advanced prostate cancer as those who didn't drink milk at all. [373] A more recent analysis of the Harvard study participants found that men with the highest calcium intake, at least 2,000 milligrams a day, had nearly double the risk of developing fatal prostate cancer as those who had the lowest intake (less than 500 milligrams per day). [374]

Dr. Tongzhang Zheng and colleagues of the department of Epidemiology and Public Health at Yale University School of Medicine, performed a population-based case-control study (601 cases and 717 controls) to evaluate the relation between diet and nutrient intakes and the risk of non-Hodgkin's lymphoma between the years 1995–2001 among Connecticut women. When the highest quartile of intake was compared with the lowest, the authors found an increased risk of non-Hodgkin's lymphoma associated with animal protein and saturated fat consumption, and no relation for vegetable protein and monounsaturated fat (found in cashews, avocado, high fat fruit, and olive) consumption. An increased risk was also observed for higher intakes of eggs and dairy products. On the other hand, a reduced risk was found for higher intakes of dietary fiber and for several fruit and vegetable items. An association between dietary intake and non-Hodgkin's lymphoma risk is biologically plausible because diets high in protein and fat may lead to altered immunocompetence, resulting in an increased risk of non-Hodgkin's lymphoma. He concluded that the antioxidant and other properties of vegetables and fruits may result in a reduced risk of non-Hodgkin's lymphoma.

Another study was conducted by Professor T. Colin Campbell, an American nutritional biochemist, known for his support for a low-fat, whole food, vegan (plant-based) diet, and the author of over 300 research papers on the subject. Campbell replicated a study done in India with his graduate students in Cornell University that showed the effect of dietary animal protein (casein) found in cow's milk on the risk of developing cancer. He exposed a group of rats to a powerful carcinogen (cancer causing agent), and then divided the group into two. One group was fed a 20% animal protein diet (casein) and the other group a 5% animal protein (casein) diet. All of the rats in the 20% group developed liver cancer or cancer precursor lesions, while not one of the rats in the 5% group did. He performed this experiment several times until he was satisfied that his results were genuine. [375] His results clearly showed that dairy animal protein intake determined liver cancer development much more than the influence of the environmental cancer promoting agent. High levels of casein consumption (20% of the diet), found in cow's milk, led to 100% increase in risk for developing liver cancer. [375]

Dairy Foods and Diabetes: The Facts

Diabetes is on a rise! There is a 62 per cent increase in people suffering from diabetes in the past decade. Figures show an increase of 17% in amputations every week due to diabetes. [376]

Insulin-dependent (Type 1 or childhood-onset) diabetes is also linked to consumption of dairy products in infancy. [377] A 2001 Finnish study of 3,000 infants with genetically increased risk for developing diabetes showed that early introduction of cow's milk increased susceptibility to Type 1 diabetes. [378] In addition, the American Academy of Pediatrics observed up to a 30% reduction in the incidence of Type 1 diabetes in infants who avoided exposure to cow's milk protein for at least the first three months of their lives. [379, 380, 381, 382, 383]

But what makes cow's milk a triggering factor? A variety of studies have reported the association between antibodies against five major proteins present in cow's milk (caseins, α-lactalbumin, γ-globulin, albumin, and hormonal constituents), and the development of Type 1 diabetes, but anti-BSA antibodies are the ones showing the highest disease specificity.

The link between cow's milk and the autoimmune process occurring in Type 1a diabetes (in genetically predisposed childhood diabetes) whereby the body mistakenly destroys the insulin-producing cells, the β-cells in the pancreas, responsible for producing insulin, the hormone that controls blood sugar levels, may be due to molecular mimicry between cow's milk proteins and β-cell proteins. Researchers identified a similarity between the amino acid sequence in cow's milk casein to the amino acid sequence on the β-cells of the pancreas, leading the body to produce antigens against its own cells causing the destruction of the insulin producing β-cells on its own pancreas. Once the β-cells are damaged, the person can no longer form insulin and becomes dependent on an outer source of insulin to survive. [384]

Dairy Foods and Cataracts: The Facts

A cataract is a progressive clouding of the lens in the eye leading to a decrease in vision. Cow's milk has also been connected to cataracts. Research shows that excessive intake of milk aggravates naphthalene-initiated cataracts, which is probably due to oxidative damage by increased levels of free radicals. [385, 386, 387]

Dairy Foods and Modern Farming Techniques: The Facts

In order to increase milk production in cows, farmers began giving them synthetic growth hormones, making cows produce a lot more milk than naturally intended. Since their bodies were not created to produce such large quantities of milk, many infections in the milk tubules occur and pus enters the milk. This warrants the need for antibiotic use. The free use of antibiotics in farm animals that provide milk, support its release it into the food chain leading to antibiotic resistant pathogens, thus rendering some antibiotics useless when we really need them.

To summarize: A high fiber, low-fat, plant-based diet with reduced levels of meat and low, or preferably no dairy products in combination with physical exercise, smoking cessation, and stress management, can not only prevent most modern day diseases, but may also reverse them. [388, 389]

Chapter 8

The Science of Epigenetics for the Prevention/Reversal of Disease and Weight Issues

"One of the first papers I wrote at the University of Wisconsin, in 1977, was on stem cells. I realized that if I changed the environment that these cells were in, I could turn the cells into bone, and if I changed the environment a bit more, they would form fat cells."

– Bruce Lipton

During my extensive research in the field of human health I have found that proper nutrition is one of the three major keys in acquiring and maintaining health, with the other keys being a positive life attitude and a healthy external environment. Quite simply, all three of these keys to health affect the environment surrounding our cells by forming either a healthy one for cells to thrive in, or a destructive one, leading to disease and early death. If we supply our cells with a healthy, nourishing environment, they will thrive and flourish. On the other hand, if we supply our cells with an unhealthy, adverse environment, they will get sick, diseased, and slowly die. In 2007, scientists

Chapter 8 - The Science of Epigenetics for the Prevention/Reversal of Disease and Weight Issues

discovered the epigenome that basically tells us that the code of life is interactive. Your DNA is *not* your destiny.The epigenome is the record of chemical changes to the DNA and histone proteins of an organism. The DNA and histone proteins are carriers of genetic information of an organism. Changes to the epigenome can result in changes to the function of our genes, however, these changes can be reversed. [390]

Unlike our DNA sequence which is largely stable within an individual, the epigenome can be dynamically altered by environmental conditions. The epigenome does not change the DNA, but it does decide how much and which genes are expressed in different cells of the body which has major effects on every aspect of our being. Gene expression is due to lifestyle!

Our body contains an estimated 37 trillion cells [391] which contain DNA, but they do not do anything with the DNA without instructions. Our genes get these instructions from the epigenome through DNA methylation or histone modifications to the DNA:

1. DNA methylation acts like a switch for gene expression, turning it on or off. Methyl groups control expression by binding to certain bases of the DNA. Some methylation modifications that regulate gene expression are heritable and can silence the expression of certain genes from one of the parents.
2. Histone modification acts like a volume knob for gene expression, turning gene expression up or down. Histones act as spools around which the DNA winds, and can determine how tightly or loosely the DNA winds around them. If they are more loosely wound around the DNA, genes will be expressed more prominently, and if they are more tightly wound around the DNA, genes are less expressed. The presence of histone marks during gene transcription indicates that the gene expression is either being prevented or modified.

Chapter 8 - The Science of Epigenetics for the Prevention/Reversal of Disease and Weight Issues

Genes are Expressed in Result to Our Lifestyle

Gene expression responds to the cells environment. Virtually any step of gene expression can be modified. [392] The DNA within our cells remains the same throughout our lives, but the epigenetic tags change throughout our lives due to different factors, and they decide which genes get expressed and which do not.

Epigenetic tags on the DNA, can be passed down to the organism's offspring.

Our diet forms the physical basis of the environment of our cells because the nutrients that come (or don't) from our food source and water supply either create a nourishing or an adverse environment for our cells.

Our attitude also affects the environment of our cells because our mind interprets the situations that surround us and how we perceive our life situations. Our body will react in accordance with our beliefs and our perception of life. How we perceive situations will translate into stress in some people, but not in others. Our cells release specific hormones and neurotransmitters in reaction to how we view these situations which will affect the environment of our cells.

Our nutrition also affects the release of hormones and other chemical messengers throughout our body therefore nutrition also has an indirect effect on the environment of our cells, as well as the direct effect of nourishing the environment of our cells with proper nutrients.

Proper nutrition, a healthy state of mind, and a natural environment low in toxins have the power to change your core health as well as any symptoms that you may be suffering from, including a larger than desired waistline and all of the common, modern day Western world diseases of which we are only too familiar. Proper nutrition and a healthy state of mind affect your health more than your DNA due to the effects on your epigenome, and this is a fact. Environment has more influence on the health of a cell than the DNA

Chapter 8 - The Science of Epigenetics for the Prevention/Reversal of Disease and Weight Issues

of that cell because dietary choices and lifestyle choices have major effects on the epigenome.

Only 10% of cancers are strictly hereditary. Hereditary cancers occur at a young age whereby the person inherits one mutant gene from their parents which predisposes them to cancer. However, for a cancer to manifest, two mutations must occur and the second mutation may result from a mitotic error during the many cell division that occur in a person's life. Hereditary cancers have a much higher incidence of multiple tumors. The remaining 90% of cancers arise sporadically from an unhealthy environment of our cells which may be lacking in nutrients or burdened with poisons and waste products.

We are not victims of our genes. Genes are potential, and not the "be all – end all" of our existence. We now know that we can consciously create our world and not just react to it. We are creators of our world, not victims to it.

In 1953, Watson and Francis Crick were the first scientists to formulate an accurate description of the DNA's complex double-helical structure. This was a great stride in the understanding of the human genome and the importance of DNA to life and health. [393] However, once they formulated the DNA description, Francis Crick suggested the theory which he called "the central dogma" of molecular biology that says that it is only one way from our DNA to our proteins that make up who we are. The meaning of "the central dogma" is that our genes are the creators of our life and we have no input. [394]

By thinking that we are made as we are from our genes, we stop caring about what we do to our bodies because we believe that we cannot change our situation. We begin to believe that disease is our destiny and become apathetic to our situation. We stop taking responsibility for our lives because we feel that we have no control over it. When this happens, people then find themselves relying on doctors and medications as a source of hope and relief.

However, it recently became clear that the concept of "the central dogma" of molecular biology is not accurate. [395]

Chapter 8 - The Science of Epigenetics for the Prevention/Reversal of Disease and Weight Issues

Yes, genes *are* blueprints that make proteins, but we now know that these blueprints can be influenced in such a way that they produce entirely different results.

Stem cells are undifferentiated biological cells that can differentiate into specialized cells and can divide (through mitosis) to produce more stem cells. [396] Stem cells act as a repair system for the body, replenishing adult tissues. Every day cells die and we replace these billions of cells that have died with new ones.

If we take stem cells and place them on a Petri dish with a cultured medium that we make as similar as possible to the fluids in the part of the body where the cells grow, the stem cell will multiply to create many of the same cells. We can then take the multiplied identical stem cells and separate them into different groups on separate petri dishes. Each group is then placed in a different culture medium. We will see that the cells will differentiate into different cells and form different tissues (muscle, fat, bone cells etc.). [397]

This clearly shows that the environment controls the destiny of the cells!

To survive in a changing world, cells have evolved mechanisms through a flexible epigenome for adjusting their biochemistry in response to signals of environmental change. [397] This allows us to adjust to changes in the world around us and to learn from our experiences. The epigenome changes in response to signals which come from inside the cell, from neighboring cells, or from our external environment. An unhealthy diet, for example, can lead to methyl groups binding to unwanted places on the genome leading to disease.

Our Lifestyle Choices Also Affect Our Future Generations Through Epigenetic Tags on Our DNA

It was also previously thought that whatever lifestyle choices we make during our lives will affect only our own health, our own waistline, and our own longevity, but they won't affect future

Chapter 8 - The Science of Epigenetics for the Prevention/Reversal of Disease and Weight Issues

generations or change our DNA. We were sure that when we had offspring, their genetic slate would be wiped clean of all of our non-beneficial lifestyle choices, and that we have no responsibility towards the health of future generations through our own choices. However, it is now known that this is not the case. Some epigenetic factors have been proven to be hereditary! It is true that some epigenetic tags are stripped off of the embryo's DNA before birth, however, now we understand that some epigenetic changes persist from generation to generation.

If our grandparents ate in an unhealthy way, some of the epigenetic changes that occurred as a result of this are passed on to future generations. This was proven in the year 2000 by a group of Swedish scientists, led by Dr. Lars Olov Bygren, a preventive-health specialist, at the Karolinska Institute in Stockholm. They examined the population of the Swedish remote town of Norrbotton in the 1800s. Norbotten is a remote area located in northern Sweden, nearly free of human life, with an average of just two people living in each square kilometer. Due to the lands' isolation, if the harvest was bad or failed completely, people nearly starved to death, and if crops were abundant, the people ate abundantly.

Dr. Bygren and his team examined the data and looked at the long-term effects of feast years and famine years on children growing up in Norrbotten in the 19th century, as well as on their children and grandchildren as well. They drew a random sample of ninety-nine individuals born in the Overkalix parish of Norrbotten in 1905 and used very precise historical records that were well maintained by the Swedish government to trace their parents and grandparents back to birth. By meticulous analysis of the agricultural records, they determined how much food had been available to the parents and grandparents when they were young. They found that conditions in the womb affected the health of the child, not only as a fetus, but also well into adulthood. They noticed that if a pregnant woman ate poorly, her child would have a significantly higher than average risk for cardiovascular disease as an adult. [398] Bygren and his colleagues

Chapter 8 - The Science of Epigenetics for the Prevention/Reversal of Disease and Weight Issues

concluded that parent's experiences early in their own lives can change the traits they pass on to their offspring.

The results of this study shows that children who enjoyed those rare, plentiful winters, and went from normal eating to gluttony in a single season, produced children and grandchildren who lived much shorter lives. Once Bygren and his team added socioeconomic variations to their research results, the difference in longevity jumped to an astonishing thirty-two years.

Simply put, the data suggested that a single winter of overeating as a youngster could initiate a biological chain of events that would lead one's *grandchildren* to die decades earlier than their peers!

Not only can we ruin our own health by our lifestyle choices, it's becoming clear that those same bad choices can also predispose our children and our children's children, even before conception, to disease and early death.

If you choose to smoke heavily or live a very sedentary lifestyle today, you will change epigenetic tags on your DNA that will not only affect you, but also the generations after you.

It is thought that autoimmune disorders previously unrecorded, and the diabetes and obesity epidemics of today are due to epigenetic changes that come from our grandparents and perhaps even their previous ancestor's lifestyle choices.

The importance of epigenetic DNA methylation in altering the physical characteristics of an organism was proven in 2003 by Duke University oncologist, Randy Jirtle, and his postdoctoral student, Robert Waterland. They conducted an experiment on mice with a uniquely regulated agouti gene; a gene that makes mice have yellow fur and a high tendency for obesity and diabetes. Jirtle's team fed one group of pregnant agouti mice a diet supplemented with methyl donors, i.e. folic acid, choline, vitamin B_{12}, and betaine, and another group of genetically identical pregnant agouti mice on a diet without these methyl donor nutrient supplements.

In the group of supplemented agouti mice, they found that the B vitamins acted as epigenetic methyl donors and caused methyl

Chapter 8 - The Science of Epigenetics for the Prevention/Reversal of Disease and Weight Issues

groups to attach more frequently to the agouti gene before they were born while still in the womb, thereby altering its expression. So without altering the genomic structure of mouse DNA, and by simply supplementing their diet with B vitamins, Jirtle and Waterland got agouti mothers to produce healthy brown mice that were of normal weight and not prone to diabetes and obesity! [399]

A subsequent study showed that the phytoestrogen genistein, found in a number of plants including fava beans, soybeans, and other legumes, [400, 401] also modified the fetal epigenome, altered the fur color, and protected the agouti offspring from obesity even though it was not capable of donating a methyl group. [402] This was followed by a study that showed that by supplementing the diet with the phytoestrogen genistein and methyl donor rich foods we could counteract detrimental epigenetic effects induced by the controversial xenobiotic chemical, Bisphenol A (BPA). [403]

In the first chapter of this book I described how the human genome is so similar to that of apes. Dr. Yoav Gilad, associate professor of human genetics at the University of Chicago, and his research team reported that up to 40% of the differences in the expression or activity patterns of genes between humans, chimpanzees, and rhesus monkeys, can be explained by epigenetic mechanisms that determine when and how a gene's DNA code is transcribed to a messenger RNA molecule to produce proteins. Dr. Gilad's team also determined that the epigenetics process of histone modification differs in the three species. In all three species, they found that transcription factor and histone modifications were identical only in 68% of regulatory elements in DNA segments that are regarded as promoter regions between apes and humans. [404, 405]

The science of epigenetics shows how important these changes are to our total being.

Judith Stern, Professor of Nutrition and Internal Medicine from the University of California at Davis, put it precisely when she said: "Genetics loads the gun, but epigenetics pulls the trigger."

Chapter 8 - The Science of Epigenetics for the Prevention/Reversal of Disease and Weight Issues

We all make lifestyle decisions that will affect our family members long after we are gone through hereditary epigenetic changes to their genome.

Parents actually have a genetic responsibility toward their children. We must guard our genome through proper life enhancing choices that we can pass onto our future generations.

I am sure that through epigenetics, and not genetics, both my sister and I were more susceptible to suffer from bulimia. We likely had epigenetic markings of starvation that led us to want to eat nonstop all of the sugar and fat-laden foods we could lay our hands on. Our maternal grandfather was a young Jewish boy raised in Germany. He was born in 1923 and was fifteen years old at the time the Second World War broke out in Germany. He was separated from his family and suffered from severe starvation and hard physical work in the three concentration camps he survived, Auschwitz, Treblinka, and Dachau. He survived the war, but surely his experiences left epigenetic tags on his DNA that were not removed from the genome passed on to my mother and then to my sister and I. My mother has suffered from weight issues all of her life due to her love for fat and sugar rich foods. Now science is showing us how we can change these epigenetic markings by choosing foods that help physically change epigenetic markings so that we are not doomed to a life of ill health and obesity.

Now, thank goodness, in most of the world, we have an almost unlimited supply of foods available readily for us, therefore we personally have the responsibility to make the right eating choices for our own health, but also for our future generations.

Even if you already have children, by teaching them proper nutrition practices and making proper lifestyle choices, you are ensuring that they and their future generations will thrive. By understanding these implications we hold responsibility for how we feed our children. Children learn best through imitation. The best way to teach them what to eat is to set a good example and explain your choices. Your children will choose to eat and to live their lives mainly by what they see you doing.

Chapter 8 - The Science of Epigenetics for the Prevention/Reversal of Disease and Weight Issues

Your choices today have heavy implications. By changing your dietary and lifestyle choices, you are certainly not only creating a better life for you and your family, but also for the future of the human race and for the world at large.

Chapter 9

Principles of Healthy Sleep

"Sleep is that golden chain that ties health and our bodies together."

— Thomas Dekker

We spend roughly a third of our lives asleep, and yet it is perhaps the least understood of all of our activities. Sleep plays an important role in the maintenance of good health. Rapid Eye Movement (REM) sleep allows for high neuronal activity and self-organization of neurons in the developing brain. Getting a good night's sleep has a direct effect on mental and physical health, as well as a person's quality of life.

Sleep and Mental Health

Sleep is an important factor in determining your mood throughout the day. If you sleep in comfortable and quiet surroundings with little stimulation to your five senses, you will sleep soundly. During sleep, your body is working to ensure healthy brain function. While you are sleeping, your brain is preparing for the next day. It's forming new neural pathways to help you support the memory of new information you have collected throughout the day as well as recalling and practicing new skills you learned while you were awake (known as consolidation).

Chapter 9 - Principles of Healthy Sleep

Studies show that a good night's sleep improves learning [406] and enhances problem-solving skills. Sleep also increases our attention span and helps us make better decisions.Dr. David M. Rapoport, associate professor at NYU Langone Medical Center, says that: "If you are trying to learn something, whether its physical or mental, you learn it to a certain point with practice, but something happens while you sleep that makes you learn it better."

A 2009 study in the Journal of Pediatrics found that children ages seven and eight who got less than eight hours of sleep a night were more likely to be hyperactive, inattentive, and impulsive. [407]

During my medical research studies at the Sakler School of Medicine at the University of Tel Aviv, I worked to support my family as an Emergency Medical Technician. This job is based on shift work and the highest paid shift is the night shift.

When my two eldest girls were spending the night at my ex-husband's house, I would work the night shift to earn as much money as I could. My concentration and mood were affected tremendously. I noticed I was eating more than usual, was falling asleep in parks while spending time with my daughters, and was more tense and angrier. I actually felt quite helpless. Being awake at night while sleeping during the day is so unnatural for us that it affects every organ in our body. Weight loss is very difficult to achieve when we are not sleeping properly. I remember that I would totally forget if I had eaten or not so I would eat again. I was totally disassociated from my body at the time. Proper sleep is a major foundation for health and weight loss. Sleep deprivation affects mental as well as physical health.

Sleep and Physical Health

Sleep helps maintain physical health. Getting enough quality sleep at the right time helps your body to function well throughout the day.

Sleep deprivation also raises the risk for many chronic health problems. [408, 409, 410]

Sleep Deprivation and Inflammation

Research indicates that people who get less than six hours of sleep have higher blood levels of inflammatory proteins than those who get more sleep. Inflammation, as I mentioned previously, is linked to heart disease, stroke, diabetes, arthritis, and premature aging. [411]

A 2010 study found that C-reactive protein, of which the levels rise in response to inflammation, was higher in people who got six or less hours of sleep. High C-reactive protein levels are associated with an increased risk for suffering from a heart attack and stroke. Sleep deprivation also triggers stress hormones such as cortisol which also contribute to heart disease and many other diseases. [412]

Data from the META-Health study (a community based Morehouse and Emory Team to Eliminate Health Disparities Study) conducted by Dr. Alanna Morris, a cardiology fellow at Emory University School of Medicine, showed that acute sleep deprivation leads to an increased production of three inflammatory hormones and to changes in blood vessel function. Individuals who reported six or fewer hours of sleep had higher levels of the following three inflammatory markers: fibrinogen, IL-6, and C-reactive protein. In particular, average C-reactive protein levels were about 25% higher in people who reported fewer than six hours of sleep compared to those reporting between six and nine hours. [413]

People whose C-reactive protein levels are in the upper third of the population (above 3 milligrams per liter) have roughly double the risk of a heart attack, compared with people with lower C-reactive protein levels, according to the American Heart Association and Centers for Disease Control and Prevention. [414, 415] Dr. Morris states that Inflammation may be one way poor sleep quality increases the risks for heart disease and stroke. [416]

Chapter 9 - Principles of Healthy Sleep

Sleep and Body Weight

Throughout childhood and puberty sleep also supports proper growth and development. Deep sleep triggers the body to release growth hormones that promotes normal growth in children and teens. This hormone also boosts muscle mass and helps in the healing and repair of cells and tissues. Sleep also plays a role in puberty and fertility by affecting hormone levels.

Sleep helps maintain a healthy balance of the hormones that make you feel hungry (ghrelin) or full (leptin), and thereby has a direct effect on the weight of an individual. When you don't get enough sleep, your levels of ghrelin, the appetite stimulating hormone, go up, and your levels of leptin, the satiety inducing hormone, go down. This makes you feel hungrier than when you are well-rested. A study found that young men who were deprived of sleep had higher levels of ghrelin and lower levels of leptin, with a corresponding increase in hunger and appetite, especially for foods rich in fat and carbohydrates. [417, 418]

People who are awake more hours have also more time to spend eating, and they do this frequently, causing weight gain. [419] Also, people who were deprived of sleep and surrounded by tasty snacks tended to snack more than when they had adequate sleep. [420] One study of Japanese workers found that those who slept fewer than six hours a night were more likely to eat out, have irregular meal patterns, and snack more than people who slept more than six hours. [421]

Researchers at the University of Chicago found that dieters who were well rested lost more fat than those who were sleep deprived. In fact, those who were sleep deprived lost more muscle mass than fat tissue. Dieters in the study also felt hungrier when they got less sleep. Actually, sleep and metabolism are controlled in the same parts of the brain. People who do not get enough sleep are more tired during the day, and consequently do less physical activity. [422]

Sleep also affects how your body reacts to insulin, the hormone that controls blood sugar levels. Sleep deficiency results in a higher than normal blood sugar level which may increase risk for type II diabetes. [423, 424]

A Stanford University study found that college basketball players who tried to sleep at least ten hours a night for seven to eight weeks significantly improved their average sprint time and had less daytime fatigue and more stamina. [425] The results of this study reflects previous findings seen in throwing darts, swimming, and weight lifting performance. [426, 427, 428]

The immune system relies on sleep to remain healthy. Ongoing sleep deficiency changes immune system function reducing immunity to common infections.

Too much or too little sleep is also associated with a shorter lifespan. In a systematic search of sixteen prospective studies from 1966-2009 which included 1,382,999 male and female participants with a follow-up range of four to twenty-five years, and 112,566 deaths, found that both too short and too long duration of sleep are significant predictors of death in prospective population studies. [429]

Sleep deficiency may also have an instant effect on our health, such as being more susceptible to car crashes if driving. It was proven that sleep deprivation has a more powerful effect on the clarity of thought and on the rate of reaction than alcohol consumption.

It is estimated that sleepiness accounts for up to 20% of crashes on monotonous roads, especially highways. [430] In 2011, the National Department of Transportation in the US estimated that drowsy driving was responsible for 1,550 fatalities and 40,000 non-fatal injuries every year. [431]

Sleep and the Quality of Life

Studies show that sleep deficiency alters activity in some parts of the brain and may predispose a person to depression, suicide, lowered motivation, and higher risk-taking behavior as well as emotional irritability. People who are sleep deficient may also have problems getting along with others. They have increased feelings of anger and impulsiveness, mood swings, and they lack motivation. (432)

Sleep deprivation affects how efficiently one works and learns. (433) Sleep deprived people take longer to finish tasks and make more mistakes.

Dr. Raymonde Jean, director of sleep medicine and associate director of critical care at St. Luke's-Roosevelt Hospital Centre in New York City, says: "If you sleep better, you can certainly live better. A good night's sleep can really help a moody person decrease their anxiety. You get more emotional stability with good sleep."

After several nights of losing sleep, even a loss of just one to two hours per night, the ability to function decreases drastically. As a result, sleep deficiency is not only harmful on a personal level, but it also can cause large scale damage. For example, sleep deficiency has played a role in human errors linked to tragic accidents, such as nuclear reactor meltdowns, sinking of large ships, as well as aviation accidents.

How Much Sleep is Enough?

The amount of sleep one needs each day changes over the course of a lifetime. Although sleep needs vary from person to person, there are general recommendations for different age groups.

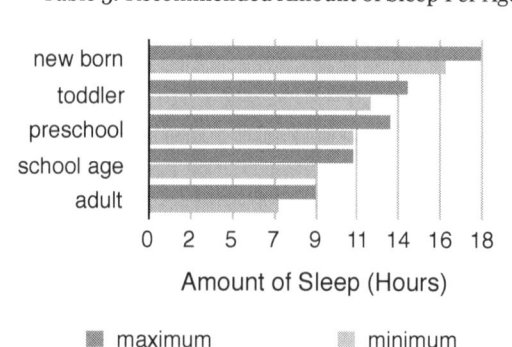

Table 5: Recommended Amount of Sleep Per Age Group

Chapter 9 - Principles of Healthy Sleep

Making up for the lack of sleep of previous days with oversleeping is never as efficient or effective as aiming for better consistency.

By setting a consistent bedtime, limiting caffeine intake late in the day, and cutting back on modern-day distractions and strong lights before bed, it is possible to increase the REM sleep time which helps reduce all of the negative effects of sleep deprivation.

What is the Best Way to Sleep?

Let's examine ape and early human sleeping patterns.

The mountain gorillas in the Virunga Volcanoes wake up with sunrise and forage in early morning (exercise), and then they may take two more rests during the day at around 10:00 am and at 1:00 pm. In the afternoon they forage (exercise) again before resting at night. When the weather is cold and grey, then they often stay longer in their nests before starting their day.

Thomas Wynn, a Professor of Anthropology at the University of Colorado, Colorado Springs, explains that the period when hominins began sleeping on the ground may have been pivotal for their cognitive development. It allowed them to spend more of the night in REM sleep, which is important for cognition and memory consolidation, (crystalizing recent memories into long-term memory). [434]

A common feature of REM sleep is muscle paralysis, which is quite impossible for apes that sleep in trees due to the many variables of uncertainty. The ape could fall off the tree or get thrown off it during the night time making deep REM sleep unlikely.

On the other hand, ground-sleeping does allow this and could have provided a cognitive boost for humans. [435]

When early hominins mastered fire, this allowed them to have an even more restful sleep because predators would have been afraid to come near the fire, and it also allowed them to achieve a constant body temperature further reducing their stress levels during the night. However, proving this theory is difficult. Kathelijne Koops from the Department of Archaeology and Anthropology, at the

Chapter 9 - Principles of Healthy Sleep

University of Cambridge, Cambridge says: "This topic is far into the realm of speculation."

Nowadays, due to round-the-clock access to technology and work schedules, an estimated 50-70 million US adults have sleep disorders. [436] Sleep problems add billions of dollars to national health care costs around the world.

There are eighty-four classifications of sleep disorders. 20-40% of all adults have insomnia during the course of any year.

However, there is evidence to show that if you do wake up in the night and later go back to get a restful sleep of enough combined sufficient hours, then you don't need to worry about sleep deprivation. In fact, nocturnal awakenings aren't abnormal at all. Some scientists concluded that they are, in fact, the natural rhythm that our body gravitates toward. According to many historians and psychiatrists, it is the compressed, continuous eight-hour sleep routine to which everyone aspires today that is unprecedented in human history.

Roger Ekirch, a sleep historian at Virginia Tech University and author of *At Day's Close: Night in Times Past*, claims that before lighting became cheap, people were accustomed to going to bed shortly after sundown, and sleeping for four hours, calling this the "first sleep," followed by a period of meditative wakefulness, and then going to back to sleep again for another four hour block called the "second sleep." During the period of meditative wakefulness some people stayed in bed, some prayed, some thought about their dreams or talked with their spouses. Others may have gotten up to do certain tasks before going back to sleep. [437]

Ekirch explained that this gave a great deal of flexibility to their nightly sleep requirements. Segmented or biphasic sleep patterns evolved to fill the long stretch of nighttime. In Africa, the darkness of night time lasted over eleven hours in the summer and over twelve hours in the winter. This is a long time to sleep. Anthropologists observe that segmented sleep continues to be the norm for many people in undeveloped parts of the world, including certain parts of Africa to this day.

Chapter 9 - Principles of Healthy Sleep

In the early '90s, psychiatrist Thomas Wehr of the National Institute of Mental Health, (a component of the U.S. Department of Health and Human Services) conducted a study on photoperiodicity (exposure to light) and its effect on sleep patterns. [438] In his study, Wehr placed a group of volunteers in an environment in which it was dark for fourteen hours of the day for a month, mimicking the days in mid-winter with shorter daylight and longer nights.

The subjects were able to sleep as much as they wanted during the experiment. During the first three weeks, the subjects slept an average of eleven hours a night. This was judged as probably a repayment for chronic sleep debt due to the modern day lifestyle. But by the fourth week, once they had caught up on their sleep, a strange thing started to happen: they began to have two sleep periods. [438]

The subjects would sleep an average of eight hours a night, but in two separate blocks. Subjects tended to sleep three to five hours in the first block and then they would awaken and spend an hour or two in quiet wakefulness before a second three to five hour sleep period. The individuals did not stress about falling back asleep, but used the time to relax. It was thus suggested that such a *biphasic* pattern of sleep is the natural or pre-historic tendency for humans. [438]

Unfortunately, no research into the natural sleeping patterns in primates in the wild was cited for comparison.

Professor of Circadian Neuroscience at Oxford, Russell Foster, states that many people wake up at night and begin to panic that they won't be getting enough sleep. "I tell them that what they are experiencing is a throwback to the bi-modal sleep pattern." [439]

For most of us, going back to the bimodal way of sleep is impossible in our current modern lifestyle. However, if you do want to regain or maintain health as well as weight loss, there is much importance in the quality and efficiency of sleep.

Good sleep is reinforced by our natural Circadian Rhythm controlled within the brain. The onset of sleep is linked to a spike in the secretion of the hormone melatonin by the brain's pineal gland, which is triggered by darkness and coordinates and reinforces sleep.

Chapter 9 - Principles of Healthy Sleep

The Circadian Rhythm may be disrupted by many situations including noise, intense exposure to light, and inconsistent bedtime hours. These confuse the Circadian Rhythm that reinforces sleepiness and sleep efficiency. Stress also leads to raised adrenalin levels which interfere with the sleeping state. Adrenaline affects the ability to fall asleep and reduces sleep efficiency, often causing frequent waking and sometimes difficulty in falling back to sleep.

But what can be done if we don't have the opportunity to sleep enough? A study investigated the effects of a thirty minute daytime nap opportunity on alertness/sleepiness. Researchers found that napping brought performance to baseline levels, and subjective sleepiness decreased significantly. It was concluded that the short nap had a clear, positive effect on alertness. [440] This effect must be similar in gorillas and this may be the reason they nap often.

Sleep Recommendations:

- Try to go to bed and wake up at the same time every day. For children, have a set bedtime schedule and a bedtime routine.
- Try to keep the same sleep schedule on weeknights and weekends. Limit the difference to no more than about an hour. Staying up late and sleeping in late on weekends will disrupt your Circadian Rhythm.
- Use the hour before bedtime for quiet time. Avoid bright artificial lights, especially blue light, such as from a TV smartphone or computer screen. The blue light emitted from these screens may signal to the brain that its time to be awake.
- Avoid heavy and/or large meals within two hours of bedtime, but small snacks are actually beneficial.
- Consume foods that improve sleep. The foods that have a direct effect on our sleep habits are foods that are rich in the hormone melatonin which is also produced by the pineal gland in our brain. Melatonin controls your circadian rhythm, and regulates hormones. As we age, production of melatonin by the pineal gland drops leading to more frequent insomnia. The best way to boost melatonin is to consume foods with naturally higher levels of

Chapter 9 - Principles of Healthy Sleep

melatonin content. Research shows that tart cherries, almonds, goji berries, raspberries, pineapples, bananas, and oranges significantly increase melatonin presence. Pineapples increased the presence of melatonin over 266% while bananas increased levels by 180%. Oranges were able to increase melatonin by approximately 47%. Melatonin also has other health benefits. Melatonin improves immune function, melatonin has anti-aging properties, and it enhances the effects of drugs used to fight cancer. I recommend improving your sleep by consuming a melatonin rich food as a snack half an hour before going to bed. The ten foods richest in melatonin include 1. Goji berries 2. Tart cherries 3. Raspberries 4. Almonds 5. Pineapples 6. Bananas 7. Oranges 8. Oats 9. Tomatoes 10. Walnuts.

- Avoid smoking at least two to three hours before bedtime. Nicotine is a stimulant.
- Avoid consumption of caffeine (including caffeinated soda, coffee, tea, and chocolate) several hours before bedtime. Caffeine is also a stimulant which may interfere with sleep. The effects of caffeine can last as long as eight hours, so a cup of coffee in the late afternoon can make it hard for you to fall asleep at night.
- Spend time out of the house in the fresh air every day. This is also especially important for babies and the elderly. Early humans used to spend their whole day outdoors. They were both healthy and brainy. It is important to get *some* fresh air a day, even if it's only twenty minutes.
- Exercise, both mental and physical, are excellent sleep enhancers if completed at least five hours before bedtime. Exercise, in addition to improving sleep, is also powerful at reducing daytime fatigue, raising metabolic rate, and improving general energy levels.
- Keep your bedroom quiet, cool, and as dark as possible. Cover all windows or use an eye cover when you sleep.
- Take a hot bath or shower, or you can use other relaxation methods before bed such as breathing techniques or meditation. I recommend a short meditation focusing on your health and weight loss goals which I've included in Chapter 15. This is a great

quietening meditation I personally use every night before falling asleep.
- Napping during the day may provide a boost in alertness and performance. However, if you have trouble falling asleep at night, limit nap times to no more than twenty minutes a day, or take them earlier in the afternoon. [441]

Chapter 10

Neuroplasticity and The Principles of a Positive Mindset

"Progress is impossible without change, and those who cannot change their minds cannot change anything."

— *George Bernard Shaw*

During the last twenty years, scientists have discovered some amazing facts about the human brain and mind. The major discoveries are in the field of neuroplasticity. Neuroplasticity reveals that our brains on the whole and our brain cells and the neural networks within our brains, have the capacity to change their connections and behavior in response to new information, sensory stimulation, development, the environment, damage, or dysfunction. [442]

The Brain is Not Static

The brain is not static, just as our DNA does not control our life as previously believed. Our brain has the ability to grow new neural connections and new brain cells, and can continually change throughout our lives. Although most neurons in the mammalian

Chapter 10 - Neuroplasticity and The Principles of a Positive Mindset

brain are formed before birth, parts of the adult brain retain the ability to grow new neurons from neural stem cells in a process known as neurogenesis (the birth of neurons).We now know, through new scientific data, that we have the ability to change every aspect of our lives and to create the life that we want to live without allowing old and non-beneficial behavioral patterns, nor our genes, to pave the path which has brought us to the life we are living today.

The brains thought patterns can be changed simply by repeatedly thinking in a certain way and by focusing ones thoughts. This allows new neural connections between brain cells to form, thereby changing the way we perceive things, thus changing our lives. This has profound implications on our ability to achieve our desires, change our habits, and achieve our livelihood. You can learn to reprogram your brain, your behaviors and emotions, so that you can achieve your goals almost automatically, and this change can happen much faster than you may believe.

Research has shown that it is the way we perceive things that will affect our behaviors and our mood. If we change our attitude about things and on what we focus upon, we can create the right mindset to create and maintain any goal, including any health and weight loss goals we may have.

In the past, I was personally dealing with major issues in all of the important fields of life. My daily living was very difficult. I was raising my two mentally disabled girls alone, I was not in a relationship, my financial situation was a total mess, and my health was terrible as I was suffering from addictions. My lawyer came to me and explained that if I didn't get my financial act together there was a possibility that my girls would be taken away from me. I then began to change my mindset about earning money and about life in general. I started to read books from the most influential self-help authors ever to have lived, and over a period of twelve months I changed my life completely around.

I researched the writer's methods and examined people that were highly successful in life in order to learn their secrets. This period involved much personal transformation for me as I delved deeply into changing irrelevant and non-useful beliefs and behaviors

Chapter 10 - Neuroplasticity and The Principles of a Positive Mindset

that I held. I found that **A PERSON IS LIMITED ONLY BY THEIR CHOICES IN LIFE!** I understood that my programmed default neural networks were constantly leading me to actions that were unsupportive of success, health and happiness in any and all fields of life. Once I learned the tools to change these thought patterns, I realized how I was personally sabotaging any possibility of success and happiness for me. I changed my thought patterns and behaviors drastically as a result of my research, and created for me the amazing life I dreamed of having, all through the science of neuroplasticity. I physically changed and reprogrammed my thought patterns by focusing them on what I wanted rather than what I didn't want. I summarized the methods I learned and used during this period in my life into my 5 book series: *"How To Achieve Success and Happiness - The 6 Principle Strategy for Creating a Successful & Happy Life"*. And through an online training program titled *"The Magic 8 Step Formula To Success, Happiness & Fulfillment. A Step-By-Step Guide To Get You Smiling & Passionate About Life Starting Now"*. Both are available on my personal development website - **Obstacle2Opportunity.com**

Now that we understand that we can change the way we behave and form new habits easily through the science of neurogenesis, it is important to understand why we behave in certain ways in the first place so that we can use behavioral science to help us achieve the life of our dreams.

By taking a glimpse at evolution, we can understand where some of our basic behaviors come from. Through this understanding, we can find ways to improve ourselves and to help us achieve our goals more easily.

In Chapter 3 I looked at evolution and how humans appeared on earth through the many evolutionary changes that have brought about the modern human being that we are today. I went into some detail of how all mammals came from a fish, which left life in the water about 350 million years ago to become a land animal. This land animal later branched off into two groups 256 million years ago, of which one group became a diverse range of reptiles and the other

Chapter 10 - Neuroplasticity and The Principles of a Positive Mindset

group became mammals. From the mammals, the *homininae* lineage appeared 8 million years ago which eventually led to modern humans. [443, 444] As we advanced to become the modern day humans, our brains developed new and more developed brain sections allowing us to think as we do today.

Some aspects of brain structure are common amongst the entire range of animal species, [445, 446] and other parts of the brain distinguish more advanced species from more primitive ones. [447]

The primitive "reptilian" brain parts, including the brain stem and the cerebellum, are reflex organs: they don't "think" – they react to situations. Whereas our higher brain parts, which make up over 90% of human brains, including the "neocortex," is where information is processed. This part of the brain found only in more developed species has the ability to think, plan, reason, to make conscious decisions, and to process language. [448]

All of our sensory organs feed the information they receive from the environment and how we perceive the environment into the primitive brain parts first before going up to higher regions of the brain that involve thinking. This is why we sometimes act before we think.

The primitive reptilian brain is programmed for our survival and protection. It is programmed to avoid fear, to protect us from danger, to keep us alive, and to bear children. Our reptilian brain cares for our survival, the survival of our offspring, and the survival of our species.

Chapter 10 - Neuroplasticity and The Principles of a Positive Mindset

Figure 15: Comparison of Vertebrate Brains – J. Arthur Thomson

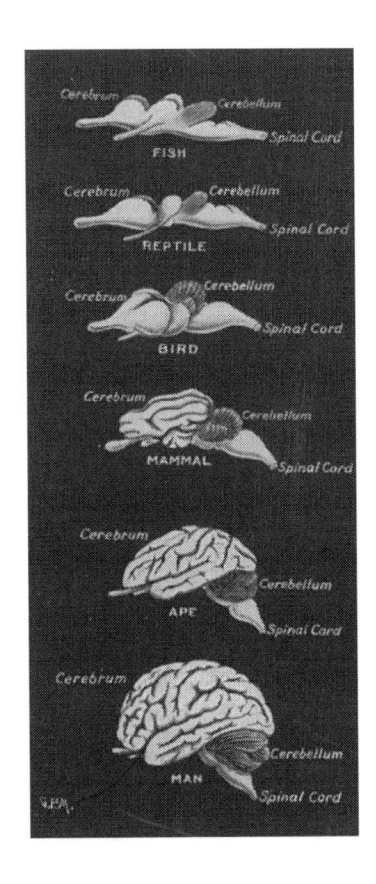

Chapter 10 - Neuroplasticity and The Principles of a Positive Mindset

Overcoming Fear of Change

The reptilian brain doesn't "like" discomfort, and it doesn't "like" to be in adventurous or new situations: It actually fears them. It prefers the common, the well-known, the easy, and the comfortable. It works to notify us of what it fears as potentially dangerous situations and things.

Due to this reflex program, *every change you decide to make in your life is going to be a challenge,* especially if the change is from something that has been ingrained within you for generations and generations like eating habits.

This is where fear comes in. We are actually born with only two fears: the fear of loud noises and the fear of falling. All other fears we have are learned from our surroundings, our own experiences, and from fears that we have recognized and accepted as real from other people whom we rely on and trust.

But what exactly is fear?

Wikipedia's definition states that "*Fear is an emotion induced by a threat perceived by the person, which causes a change in brain and organ function and ultimately a change in behavior, such as running away, hiding or freezing from traumatic events. Fear may occur in response to a specific stimulus happening in the present, or to a future situation, which is perceived as risk to health or life, status, power, security, wealth or anything held valuable. The fear response arises from the perception of danger.*" [449]

The fear of discomfort of any sort doesn't mean that the discomfort *will* in fact happen, only that it *may* happen.

Fear comes knocking on our door every time we do something or are confronted with something new. But if we don't take any new actions in our life nor change our choices to better ones than our parents perhaps did or our grandparents made, then we are not developing and becoming any better than what we are today.

We must leave our comfort zone to make our lives better and more worthy, and this is not easy, thanks to our reptilian brain. We will always have that little voice inside our heads naysaying our new path. This will happen every single time we do something that we want, but have not tried before, but this can be changed by using the understandings learned from neuroplasticity.

Raising Your Chances of Succeeding At Dieting

To lower the chance that we will behave in reaction (rather than in response) to any new or difficult situation, we must lower our instinctive reaction of fight or flight mechanism that comes from our reptilian brain.

So how do we do this?

We can do this by following these four steps:

1. Any change in lifestyle habits leads to the onset of fear and worry for many different reasons. You can control your thoughts and direct them in a way that will lead to an increase in your self-esteem and not in a way that will decrease it. Fear comes when we perceive the anticipation discomfort of any sort. When you are anticipating discomfort, meet the discomfort back with something that will cause you comfort and pleasure and raise your self-esteem. For example, let's say you are trying to reduce your sugar and fat intake and you are used to eating these types of foods. You see them on every corner you turn. You will feel discomfort from not being "allowed" to eat them on your new lifestyle plan. To stop this feeling of discomfort, you have to remind yourself of something that this lifestyle plan will lead you to that will give you great pleasure.

It is important that the pleasure you are reminding yourself of must be of greater pleasure when achieved and much greater comfort than the one you will feel by consuming these foods. You can remind yourself of how great you will look and feel. You can remind yourself of how healthy you will be. You can remind yourself of

Chapter 10 - Neuroplasticity and The Principles of a Positive Mindset

animal suffering whenever you choose to consume animal products and how pleasurable it feels not to take part in animal cruelty. You can remind yourself what you will be able to do once you have reached your goals and how these changes will bring you great pleasure. But the most powerful stimulant is when you have a reason that is perceived as life or death for you, meaning that you know that living without this in your life would make you very unhappy or even miserable.

You know what will give you greater comfort and pleasure than consuming the food itself.

Visualize in your mind a pleasurable picture of you reaching your end goal. I know this is not easy, but this is the basis of success in any and every field.

Remember that avoiding discomfort is the top priority of the reptilian brain, so you will need to identify something that will lead to greater pleasure and be attractive enough for you to overwhelm the reptilian brain programming to get you to do the right thing at the right time to help you reach your goal.

Here's an example from my life. I have healed myself from cancer by going on a diet that was somewhat new for me, and it was not easy to make all these changes very quickly.

Now for me not to fall victim to eating the unhealthy foods that I was used to, I had to remind myself that I want to lead a long and healthy life, not have a recurrence of cancer, and be strong and energetic to raise my four daughters. The pleasure of living a healthy, long life with my family gives me more comfort and pleasure than the short term benefits I would get from eating the cakes, pies, cookies, etc.

Know what is pleasurable enough for you. Visualize in your mind a picture of you reaching your end goal.

This is your true goal, not the number of pounds/kgs that you desire to lose. Remind yourself of your goal whenever you are encountered by any discomfort. This change of mindset will help you to achieve your pleasurable goal.

Chapter 10 - Neuroplasticity and The Principles of a Positive Mindset

2. When you do take action towards your goal, do it in small steps that won't overwhelm you and trigger the reptilian brain to fight against your efforts.

You must step out of your comfort zone in order to get to somewhere better, but make sure you do it in *small steps* so as not to overwhelm yourself. Taking small steps over a longer period of time rather than taking an "all or nothing" approach will work far better in bringing about change in your life. In Chapter 16, you will be provided with different weekly schedules and plans you can use to take on a new, more positive lifestyle habit every week.

By taking on change gradually, you won't enter a panicky state. You will remain calm and in control because you are tricking your mind to think that not too much has changed and therefore not too much is at risk.

It is like the French story of the frog. The French love to eat frog soup, but the cook would complain that the frog would jump out of the pot if placed in boiling water. Another cook suggested to him to place the frog in cold water and slowly heat the water until it boiled. This way the frog wouldn't jump out and would slowly cook to make a good frog soup.

This story would be quite horrendous if it were true, but the moral is that small changes are not as painful as drastic changes, and will not make us immediately run away or quit our efforts.

I even recommend not telling people around you that you are on some new kind of dietary program as this will put too much pressure on you from the beginning. Keep this information to yourself until the changes are coming on smoothly and you feel more in control of your health, your food choices, and your weight.

3. Do not focus only on your end result (the weight you want to lose). Instead focus on both your pleasurable end goal that you set in the first step for success, and on your weekly action plan that you will receive in Chapter 16. This reduces the pressure on you and allows you to do things in a more relaxed and controlled way. Follow these weekly plans according to the simple instructions given in Chapter 16. These will ensure you reach your desired end goal.

By not focusing on the end result, not weighing yourself many times a day, taking tests too often, and instead focusing on your goals and how you are doing in regard to the healthy lifestyle weekly plans, you are placing yourself in control rather than placing results in control. If you persist with the right actions, you will surely reach your goal – there is no doubt about it. Even if it takes longer than you expected, the time factor is unimportant. The main thing is that you will reach your desires, and you will certainly reach them even if you only take on 75% of the suggestions in this diet. By holding on to the steering wheel of your life and taking control by focusing on actions rather than results, simply doing the actions you will boost your self-esteem and surely reach your goal smoothly and easily.

4. The last step involves making sure that when you set a goal for yourself, it is at least 15-20% more than that which you wish to achieve. For example, if I plan to lose 8 kg (16 lb.) of weight, or I wish to get my cholesterol down to 200 mg/dl, then I should create a goal that is 15-20% higher than my original desire. Instead of creating a goal of losing only 8 kg (16 lb.), I should aim to achieve a weight loss of 9 to 10 kg (20 lb.), or getting my cholesterol down to 170mg/dl.

The reason for this is that if you miss one of the steps or recommendations listed in this diet, you may begin to believe that your goal is no longer within your reach. This will activate your primitive reptilian brain to go into survival mode, preventing you from leaving your comfort zone and achieving your goal at all.

Write down at least two action plans of how you intend to reach your goal. I have included an action plan recommendations in Chapter 16 of this book. You can follow it or you can create one of your own following the instructions in Chapter 16.

As the famous quote by Susan Jeffers goes, "Feel the fear, but do it anyway," by doing this, you will have made the biggest difference in your ability to achieve your goals, because you WILL

Chapter 10 - Neuroplasticity and The Principles of a Positive Mindset

come to see that after overcoming your fears, it was not as bad as you thought it would be after all. You will begin to believe in your abilities and see that you can succeed. This increases your self-esteem and proves to yourself that you can achieve your goals.

One excellent way to increase your self-esteem is to get some "feel good" hormones pumping in your blood stream by committing to regular physical activity. Exercise triggers an overall positive feeling similar to that of the drug morphine because your body releases chemicals called endorphins, a combination of *endo* and *orphin*; two shortened forms of the words *endogenous* and *morphine,* intended to mean "a morphine-like substance originating from within the body." [450] These endorphins interact with the receptors in your brain that reduce your perception of pain, fear, and worry.

The feeling after an endurance workout is described as euphoric, sometimes also called the "runner's high."

Exercise increases the production of brain derived neurotrophic factor (BDNF), a member of brain growth factors. [451] BDNF is one of the most active brain growth factors. [452, 453, 454] BDNF acts on specific neurons supporting their survival and encouraging new growth (neurogenesis) and differentiation of neurons and synapses. [455, 456] In the brain, BDNF is active in the areas vital to learning, long-term memory, [457] and higher thinking. [458]

There are so many other benefits to exercise due to the reason that we were built to be physically active. The modern lifestyle has allowed us to become so sedentary through the technological advances that have brought us food, heat, clean water, and shelter so easily without us having to physically care for these needs. But physiologically, our bodies have not changed much in the short period that all of these advances have become available to almost all humans alive today.

If we want to maintain our health and lead a healthy, pain-free life that is not dependent on medications, then we must go by the laws of nature and eat a diet that our bodies were intended for and to remain physically active. [459, 460]

Chapter 10 - Neuroplasticity and The Principles of a Positive Mindset

Regular physical activity has been proven to:
- Reduce stress and anxiety. [461]
- Reduce feelings of depression. [461]
- Increase self-esteem and boosts confidence. [462]
- Improve sleep because of the sedative effects endorphins produce after exercise.
- Strengthen heart muscle tissue.
- Increase energy levels.
- Lower blood pressure. [463]
- Change the cholesterol profile by increasing high-density lipoprotein (HDL), and decreasing triglyceride levels. [464]
- Improve the way you move by increasing coordination, improving muscle tone and strength and boosting endurance thereby reducing falls and preventing fractures.
- Strengthening and increasing bone mass because physical activity puts stress on the bones and causes them to retain and up to a certain age even gain density. Cells within the bone can sense physical stress and respond to it by making the bone stronger and denser.
- Reduce body fat, because when you engage in physical activity, you burn more calories, [465, 466] even as you rest, by raising the body's resting metabolic rate (RMR).
- Makes you look better.
- Helps you live longer. [467]

In fact, regular physical activity has been proven to help prevent or treat such a wide range of health disorders, including heart disease, stroke, Type 2 diabetes, metabolic disease, arthritis, osteoporosis, depression, and some types of cancer, [459, 463, 468, 469, 470] that it would be ridiculous not to take part in it.

Regular physical activity is also reported to decrease inflammatory markers, [471, 472, 473] responsible for many of today's ailments.

More on physical activity will be discussed in the next chapter.

Chapter 11

An Evolutionary Approach To Physical Activity Needs

"The medical literature tells us that the most effective ways to reduce the risk of heart disease, cancer, stroke, diabetes, Alzheimer's, and many more problems are through healthy diet and exercise. Our bodies have evolved to move, yet we now use the energy in oil instead of muscles to do our work."

— David Suzuki

      Like all species, human genes were shaped by environmental pressures over millions of years of evolution.

      We have optimal exercise patterns that suit our bodies best as we are and will keep us healthy and fit. It is important to understand the evolutionary changes that occurred and how they influence our health in today's modern society.

      The first hominins to become erect, bipedal with a striding gait, appear in the fossil record around 3.5 million years ago. [474, 475, 476, 477, 478, 479, 480, 481, 482] These adaptations are quite different from

Chapter 11 - An Evolutionary Approach To Physical Activity Needs

other mammals. [483] We are ideally suited for walking in a pendular motion. This method of movement resulted in enough energy saving to have produced a selective genetical advantage. [484, 485, 486] Man is one of the best long distance walkers and runners among cursorial mammals (mammals specifically adapted to run fast or far across open spaces). Game animals are faster over shorter distances, but they have less endurance than man. [487]

Many scientists claimed that early hunters succeeded in running down their prey simply by sheer endurance until the animal collapsed of exhaustion. [488] This is due to adequate thermal regulation that humans possess which allows us to run for extended periods. Humans thermoregulate their rising body temperatures during physical exercise by sweating rather than by panting.

This has advantages and disadvantages. Sweating, as opposed to panting for heat reduction, allows us to run and breathe at the same time, and to keep body temperature lower in hot conditions. On the other hand, panting animals lose less salt while running, become less hot in hotter environments, but cannot run for long distances.

The cost of transport of a walking human is minimized at speeds of 5 kph (3 mph). When running, the speed does not define the energetic cost of running, meaning if you run faster, the energy expenditure will not be very different from running at slower speeds. This is because breathing frequency does not depend on the frequency of stride. Humans can vary their breathing frequency relative to stride frequency, something a panting animal cannot do. [489]

Humans are the highest sweating species. [490, 491] This is due to our relative lack of hair. Bare skin increases the rate at which sweat evaporates from its surface thereby increasing cooling efficacy in the sunny savanna environments. [492, 493] This exceptional capacity hominins had for heat dissipation gave them an edge over other animals living on the savanna.

Chapter 11 - An Evolutionary Approach To Physical Activity Needs

The ability to run long distances without overheating had enough survival advantages for human genetic selection by helping them escape from predators in the blazing sun, locating food and water sources, and transporting food, children, and other objects while walking. Being bipedal allowed hominins to move out of the diminishing forests due to changing weather conditions quite easily, especially since there was much competition over food sources in those forests. Hominins then began adapting to life on the savanna where food was more dispersed, but where they had little competition over it. [494]

Until the agricultural revolution, around 10,000 years ago, all hominins lived a hunter-gatherer lifestyle, roaming the land foraging for food with regular daily long distance walking or running and some strength building activities. Our genetic makeup is built to move and to exercise. Millions of years of evolution cannot be overcome by a few hundred years of a sedentary lifestyle. Since ancient times we were being regularly physically active and living in weather conditions that required a minimal state of fitness to survive. The present day sedentary lifestyle has led to epidemics among humans in modern society that were previously non-existent in ancient societies.

How does exercise help prevent modern day diseases?

Exercise enhances glucose uptake by skeletal muscles and long distance exercise increases skeletal muscle insulin sensitivity and reduces plasma insulin levels. [495, 496] In response to glucose load, people who regularly exercise secrete less insulin and have lower peak plasma glucose levels than do sedentary people. [497] This has been proven to help prevent the onset of diabetes, vascular diseases, and high blood pressure.

Running does have a high energetic cost for humans and this was overcome through a diet rich in carbohydrates. Having a regular source of high carbohydrate food doubles muscle glycogen and enhances endurance in humans. [498, 499] On the contrary, a diet rich in protein and fats decreases muscle glycogen, the energy storage molecule, and prematurely depletes glycogen stores during exercise. [500]

Chapter 11 - An Evolutionary Approach To Physical Activity Needs

It is well accepted among anthropologists that hunting was not a major hominin activity before the mid Pleistocene epoch, around 200,000 years ago, at the same time that clear evidence of cooking was found. However, persistence hunting could have played a role in the obtainment of meat for food consumption in small amounts beforehand.

Walking was used for migration, but running was required for escaping predators in the hot sun while carrying children and objects of importance, and perhaps for running down prey animals in the hot daytime, a time when animals would normally be resting. This certainly gave humans an edge over other animals and could have provided strong selection for increased intelligence, group cooperation, and precise communication. [501]

Furthermore, as mentioned in the previous chapter, evidence shows that brain growth factors including BDNF (Brain Derived Neurotrophic Factor) increases with sustained exercise. These brain growth factors help to support the survival of existing neurons and encourage the growth and differentiation of new neurons and synapses. [502, 503] Physical activity also made us smarter.

Physical activity helps us sleep better, making us calmer and overall happier. When I wanted to add physical activity to my daily schedule I bought a treadmill. But because I love running outside, I hardly used this machine. Then one day I was sitting on the floor playing with my mentally challenged and epileptic girls and the machine caught my eye. I decided to try and let my daughters take a walk on it. I played dance music in the background and persuaded them to get on the machine. They both have spastic legs so at first I put the machine on 2 km/hour speed. After their leg muscles warmed up I noticed that I could raise the speed and they could keep up. They actually loved it, and from that day on for the next two years they were on the treadmill for thirty minutes three times a week. They loved it! Their fitness improved so much that they were actually running on it. If you knew my daughters, you would be very surprised. During this time, their epileptic seizures dramatically decreased in number and they slept for longer periods of time at night. The only reason we had to stop was because when we moved from our house to an apartment building, the neighbor's below us complained about the noise.

Physical activity along with a healthy diet has tremendous potential to heal, for this is how we are intended to live.

In the next section of this book I will help you put all of the information you received in the previous chapters together to form ***The Guerrilla Diet and Lifestyle Program*** which will help you to reach your ideal weight and health in the fastest, most direct path.

SECTION 2

The Guerrilla Diet & Lifestyle Program Guidelines

Chapter 12

The Guerrilla Diet & Lifestyle Program – Introduction

"Change will not come if we wait for some other person or some other time. We are the ones we've been waiting for. We are the change that we seek."

– Barack Obama

Now you have all of the information you need to encourage you to begin the program. All of the benefits of ***The Guerrilla Diet Lifestyle Program*** have been detailed before you in the previous eleven chapters. Now it is time to put it all together and get your butt in gear to finally begin the diet and lifestyle program.

When we are born we were given our bodies, our health, and brains for free. Perhaps this is the reason why we so often take them for granted. We have been given these wonderful precious and priceless gifts as well as the amazing opportunity to be in this world, enjoy it, and influence others with our uniqueness. To do this to the best of our capabilities, we must be in good health. To

Chapter 12 - The Guerrilla Diet & Lifestyle Program – Introduction

maintain our health, we were given land on this planet, and the land can, and does, supply all of our nutritional requirements naturally. When we combine the earth's gifts along with the maintenance of an active lifestyle, conserving good relationships, and contributing to others in our unique and special way, we have the keys to our happiness and prosperity.

They are all free, they are all within our reach, and we are all capable of achieving these desires if we follow our true nature. In fact, being healthy is our birthright. Now is the time to utilize the knowledge you have gained through reading this book into your daily life style.

Our body ceaselessly removes toxins, pathogens, and unhealthy cells from our system. It is constantly working to keep us healthy and fit. It is the endless amount of toxins that we allow to enter our bodies that detract from our body's ability to maintain the health we deserve.

Obesity and overeating are learned conditions. They are learned at home since school doesn't teach us much about health and nutrition.

By reading the first two-thirds of this book, you have all the knowledge you need in order to succeed and achieve the health and beauty you deserve. But advice alone is of no use if you do not combine it with action.

It is important to understand that you are starting a marathon now and not a sprint. By reading the first eleven chapters of this book, you will have prepared yourself for this marathon run. Now you are ready to begin. This is the moment you have planned, practiced, and learned for earlier. It also helps to know that within two to three months of starting this program, the cravings for fats and sugars will mostly dissipate.

Please don't fuss about your weight. By taking the right steps and doing the right actions, the perfect weight will come naturally to you in due time. Remember, just as you didn't put the weight on in a day, don't expect it to come off in one.

Take a deep breath and let's begin to take action.

The First Action Step

First, you will need to eliminate any distractions you may have that keep you from achieving your desire, for example, if your freezer is filled with ice cream and your cupboards are filled with cakes and cookies, these will distract you on your path to optimal health and weight loss so it is best to eliminate them before you begin.

In the following chapter you will receive all of the information to understand which foods have the potential to secure health and weight loss and which don't. Once you go through the list and understanding which foods are non-beneficial to your health, go into your kitchen cabinets and remove all of the foods that are not providing you with value. You can do the same in your refrigerator and your freezer. This is not an easy step, I know, but if you want to change, you are going to have to do it at some point, so why not just start now?

Remove everything that has no value for where you desire to be in life.

The Second Action Step

Now that you have removed all of the obstacles from your way, it is time to put in the new, good things that will act as substitutes and replace your previous bad choices. After reading the first eleven chapters and the following chapter, you will completely understand which foods will benefit your health and weight loss goals.

After understanding which foods are right for you, go to a health food supermarket or your local farmers market and stock up on healthy, valuable foods, and choose options that you think you will love to eat. To do this more easily, I have supplied you with a simple recommended shopping list in Chapter 14.

Chapter 13

So, What Should We Eat... and Why?

"Tell me what you eat, and I will tell you who you are."

— Jean Anthelme Brillat-Savarin

In this chapter I have put together clear and practical advice based on the background research supplied in Section 1 of this book. This will provide you with simple guidelines for proper eating practices that will help you easily create a nourishing environment for your cells and lead you on the path to lasting health and easy weight loss.

I used to be like most people who do not have a clue as to what is proper nutrition. I was so confused with all of the information taught in different schools that at one point I felt a complete disbelief with the whole agenda of nutrition, even though I had studied it extensively at university and in alternative colleges. The information I received from my university studies in medicine and nutrition was, at times, completely contradictory to what I had learned when studying alternative nutrition. I did not have the knowledge, even though I was well educated in the field of nutrition and health, as to what food choices I should make to achieve my perfect weight as well as to maintain optimum health and vitality. I also did not fully grasp

Chapter 13 - So, What Should We Eat... and Why?

the concept that the key to my lasting health and wellness lay in my own hands through my own choices.

Most of us, including myself at the time, feed on advertisements as to what we should consume for our health, but unfortunately the media sometimes hides the truth and seeks to sell products to people in order to gain monetary benefit with no real concern for human health, from the companies that pay them hefty advertising fees.

Often the foods we consume are exactly the opposite foods that we should be eating for our dream waistline and our health. As we saw in the previous chapters, our diet also has repercussions on our future generations and the health of our planet as a whole.

Today, pharmaceutical companies sell us medications to treat certain symptoms of disease, but these medications have no influence on the causes of our problems, nor on our health as a whole, and governments around the world maintain the economic interest of the medical establishment in mind often before considering the health ramifications on humans.

So the question stands: which foods are we meant to consume to promote our health, beauty, and longevity? In this book we have examined the research behind the ultimate diet for human consumption for health, longevity, and vitality from different scientific aspects including evolution, zoology, archeology, genetics, medicine, and, of course, nutrition. When putting these sciences together with some good old common sense, the ultimate diet for human consumption and lifestyle program quickly emerges. This diet and lifestyle program have now been proven to provide people with a good looking, good feeling, healthy, energized body, while caring for our planet.

Here is The Guerrilla Diet and Lifestyle Program "recipe" for success:

Chapter 13 - So, What Should We Eat... and Why?

Dietary Guidelines

1. Consume foods with low energy density.
2. Consume foods that will not cause an inflammatory response.
3. Consume seasonal foods (foods grown according to their natural season).
4. Consume local foods.
5. Consume natural foods, cooked or raw.
6. Consume foods that will not burden the body with toxins.
7. Consume foods rich in minerals.
8. Consume foods rich in fiber to increase digestion rate and waste/toxin removal rate.
9. Consume foods low in animal protein.
10. Consume foods rich in fatty acid precursors such as kale and green leaves.
11. Consume foods that prevent calcium loss.
12. Consume foods rich in both calcium and magnesium.
13. Consume foods rich in methyl donors.
14. Consume foods rich in prebiotics for a healthy gut microbiome.
15. Get sufficient vitamin D.
16. During the day consume foods regularly so as to avoid strong feelings of hunger. During the night go on an intermittent fast of 12 hours.

After going over these guidelines in detail in this chapter, I will supply you with specific recommendations for vascular disease patients, for diabetes patients, for times of menstruation and pregnancy, for elite athletes, for living with children, and more.

Now let's take a closer look into each dietary guideline.

Chapter 13 - So, What Should We Eat... and Why?

1. Consume Foods with Low Energy Density

Filling up on low energy density foods is the best way to lose weight and support health according to a recent literature review of seventeen studies in adults, and six cohort studies in children and adolescents. They found strong and consistent evidence in adults that dietary patterns relatively low in energy density improve weight loss and weight maintenance. Consuming diets lower in energy density may be an effective strategy for managing body weight. (504) So how do we use this recommendation in our daily life? By choosing foods that contain the same amount of nutrients, but supply less energy in the form of calories. Diets higher in low energy density foods can be achieved by increasing consumption of fruit and vegetables and reducing fat intake. (505, 506) By choosing fresh fruits or dehydrated fruits rather than dried fruits, and by choosing fresh or boiled vegetables instead of fried versions, we can easily achieve this recommendation.

For example, 1/2 a cup of grapes contains 110 calories, 0.2g fat, 29 g carbohydrates and 1.1 g protein, compared to 434 calories, 0.7 g fat, 115 g carbohydrates and 4.45 g protein in 1/2 a cup of raisins.

A 100g serving of boiled potatoes contains 103 calories, 2.2g fat, 19.2 g carbohydrates and 1.8 g protein, compared to 319 calories, 17 g fat, 37 g carbohydrates and 3.7 g protein in 100g of fried potatoes.

By eating more fresh foods, we reduce energy density while receiving the same amount of nutrients if not more.

2. Consume Foods That Will Not Cause an Inflammatory Response

Heart disease, cancer, Alzheimer's, and acne, are just some of the possible consequences of too much inflammation in the body. Our bodies depend on the inflammatory process to help us fight off infections by eliminating the initial cause of cell injury. The purpose

Chapter 13 - So, What Should We Eat... and Why?

of inflammation is to clear out injured cells and tissues damaged from an exterior insult and to heal injuries, but when inflammation is not actively terminated when no longer needed, it may get out of control and become chronic and harmful to the body, leading to more extensive tissue and cellular destruction. [507]

The Western diet is known to contain many pro-inflammatory foods that are well known to donate their share to chronic, low-grade inflammation. Pro-inflammatory foods promote cytokine and eicosanoid production. They are released by cells and affect the behavior of other cells. They engage in complex control over many bodily systems including inflammation or immunity. Anti-inflammatory drugs such as aspirin and other non-steroidal anti-inflammatory drugs such as Ibuprofen act by down-regulating eicosanoid synthesis. However, by significantly reducing the amount of pro inflammatory foods consumed, we achieve similar results as taking these medications.

Pro-inflammatory foods include highly processed or refined foods. Processed or refined foods are not assimilated by the body. They cannot fulfil the body's nutritional needs and therefore they just burden the body with excess toxins.

Pro-inflammatory foods fall into the following four groups:
1. Processed foods from animal origin:
    (1) Salami/cured ham
    (2) Sausages
    (3) Pastrami
    (4) Commercial cheeses
2. Foods with a high glycemic index:
    (1) Sugar
    (2) Honey
    (3) Agave
    (4) Alcohol
3. Foods containing little or no fiber:
    (1) Fruit juices
    (2) White rice
    (3) White flours
    (4) Processed oils

4. Foods high in saturated, hydrogenated, trans fats and omega-6 (ω-6) fatty acids:
    (1) Cakes, cookies, muffins, donuts
    (2) Pie crusts, pizza dough, cake mixes
    (3) Margarine, vegetable shortening
    (4) Milk and chocolate powder drink mixes
    (5) French fries
    (6) Processed biscuits and crackers
    (7) Packaged chips/crisps
    (8) Candy and chocolate bars
    (9) Packaged popcorn
    (10) Some frozen meals

Try to completely avoid the foods on the above list.

3. Consume Seasonal Foods (Foods Grown According to Their Natural Season)

Eating seasonally is important and carries with it many benefits to your health, to the planets health, and to your wallet.

Firstly, eating seasonal foods increases the wealth of nutrients in the food itself. Foods grown out of season are not as rich in nutrients as foods that are grown in season. Foods eaten in season are also cheaper because they are at the peak of their supply and because they do not need greenhouses to be built in order to keep them safe from the weather. Seasonal foods are also tastier than foods grown out of season. The flavors are stronger and more developed, the textures are as they were meant to be, and they are tasty even when eaten in their natural state. Foods grown out of season tend to undergo chemical washes and wax coatings in order to keep them looking good. Some non-seasonal foods are transported from the other side of the world, from where they are *in* season to where they are not. These foods are usually picked before the peak of their flavor in order to survive the long trip, or they are allowed to mature as they travel. As a result, they're much more expensive because of the time, distance, energy expenses, and the sheer number of people involved in the transport process that need to be paid for getting those food items to you. These foods are much less nutritious since they lose vital nutrients during their journey. By eating seasonal foods, you are sparing the world fuel wastage, environmental damage, and are supplying yourself with cheaper, more nutritious and better tasting food.

In the US, there is a wonderful website that shows all the seasonal foods by state and month which is great because of the diversity between states. You can access it here:

Seasonal Food Guide US: **http://goo.gl/OiO5NN**

On the following pages I have included a chart of foods that are in season in the mid-European countries, including the UK, France, Germany, Holland, Romania, to name a few. In the blackened months the foods are in season and in the grey months, the foods are just entering their season. It is best to consume foods grown during the blackened months.

Chapter 13 - So, What Should We Eat... and Why?

Seasonal Food Guide For European Countries

Seasonal Food Guide For European Countries

	Jan	Fe	Mar	Apr	May	Jun	Jul	Aug	Sep	Oct	Nov	Dec
Apple	■	■							■	■	■	■
Apricot					■	■	■	■	■			
Asparagus					▨	■						
Aubergine					▨	■	■	■	■	■		
Banana	■	■	■	■	■	■	■	■	■	■	■	■
Basil						▨	■	■				
Beetroot	■							■	■	■	■	■
Blackberry						▨	■	■	■			
Black Currants					▨	■	■					
Bramley apple	■	■	■								▨	■
Broad beans					▨	■	■	■				
Broccoli						▨	■	■	■			
Brussels sprouts	■	■	■							■	■	■
Cabbage	■	■	■	■	■	■	■	■	■	■	■	■
Carrot					▨	■	■	■	■	■		
Cauliflower	■	■	■	■							▨	
Celery	■	■					▨	■	■	■	■	■

Chapter 13 - So, What Should We Eat... and Why?

Seasonal Food Guide For European Countries

	Jan	Fe	Mar	Apr	May	Jun	Jul	Aug	Sep	Oct	Nov	Dec
Celery root	■	■	■	■					■	■	■	■
Cherry						▨	■					
Chervil				■	■	■	■	■	■			
Chestnut	■								▨			
Chicory	■	■	■									
Clementine	■	■									■	■
Cranberry										■	■	■
Cucumber		▨	■	■	■	■	■	■	■	■		
Date	■									▨	■	
Fennel						■	■	■	■	■		
Fig								▨	■	■		
Garlic						▨	■	■	■	■		
Globe artichoke					▨	■	■	■	■	■	■	
Gooseberry					▨	■	■	■	■			
Grapefruit	■	■	■	■	■							■
Green onion				■	■	■	■	■				

Chapter 13 - So, What Should We Eat... and Why?

Seasonal Food Guide For European Countries

	Jan	Fe	Mar	Apr	May	Jun	Jul	Aug	Sep	Oct	Nov	Dec
Jerusalem artichoke	■	■	■							▨	■	■
Kale	■	■							▨	■	■	■
Kohlrabi							▨	■	■	■	■	
Leek	■	■	■						■	■	■	■
Lemon	■	■	■									
Lettuce				▨	■	■	■	■	■	■	■	■
Mint					■	■	■	■	■			
Nectarine					■	■	■	■	■			
New potatoes				■	■	■	■					
Onion	■	■	■	■					■	■	■	■
Orange	■	■	■									
Pak choi	■	■	■	■	■	■	■	■	■	■	■	■
Parsnip	■	■	■							■	■	■
Peach							▨	■	■			
Pear	■									■	■	■
Peas				▨	■	■	■	■	■			
Pepper		▨	■	■	■	■	■	■	■			
Plum								▨	■	■		

Chapter 13 - So, What Should We Eat... and Why?

Seasonal Food Guide For European Countries

	Jan	Fe	Mar	Apr	May	Jun	Jul	Aug	Sep	Oct	Nov	Dec
Pomegranate	■	■	■	■	■	■	■	■	■	■	■	■
Potato			▓	■	■	■	■	■				
Pumpkin									▓	■	■	■
Quince									▓	■	■	■
Radicchio	■	■	■	■	■	■	■	■	■	■	■	■
Radish			▓	■	■	■	■	■	■	■		
Raspberry					▓	■	■	■	■			
Redcurrant						▓	■	■	■			
Rhubarb	■	■	■	■	■	■						
Runner bean							■	■	■	■	■	
Spinach			▓	■	■	■	■	■	■	■		
Spring greens				■	■	■	■					
Spring onion	■	■	■	■	■	■	■	■	■	■	■	■
Strawberry					▓	■	■	■	■			
Swede	■	■								▓	■	■
Sweet potato	■	■	■							■	■	■
Sweetcorn								▓	■	▓		

Chapter 13 - So, What Should We Eat... and Why?

Seasonal Food Guide For European Countries

	Jan	Fe	Mar	Apr	May	Jun	Jul	Aug	Sep	Oct	Nov	Dec
Swiss chard												
Tomato												
Turnip												
Watercress												
Watermelon												
Zucchini												

4. Consume Local Foods

As I mentioned in the previous recommendation, foods also lose nutrients during their long trip to your local supermarket. For example, spinach and green beans lose two-thirds of their vitamin C within a week of harvest. Furthermore, during their trip to your local grocery shop, non-local foods are refrigerated, not allowing the food to mature as they would in their natural habitat.

Buying foods in farmers markets is the best way to support the local farmers who nurture their soils and sustainably manage their land. Modern commercial farming, with its focus on quantity over quality, reduces soil quality, providing us with consistently less nutritious foods. This also saves fossil fuels by saving transport around the globe.

Another benefit of eating local foods is that farmers don't have to select crops to sell based on their durability, shelf life, or yield. Instead, they can choose crop varieties for traits including taste, vitamin content, and color. The farmer who grows and sells them at the market can sometimes also give advice on how to cook these foods, thereby allowing people to try new items that they would have never bought otherwise.

5. Consume Natural Foods: Cooked or Raw

In other words, eat foods that you can imagine how they were grown or that you can grow in your own backyard if this was your desire. These foods include all vegetables, all fruits, all nuts, seeds, legumes, underground storage organs, natural honey, and all whole unprocessed grains, and naturally grown animals if you wish.

Natural foods which are in their "as close to natural" state are the best bet for keeping yourself healthy and well-nourished. When the body is well-nourished, you will see that you tend to eat less food and you will naturally find yourself consuming only what you need. When the body has its nutrients supplied there are fewer cravings for processed, high calorie, sugar, and fat rich foods that are the leading cause of obesity in our times. The health of people consuming a modern Western world diet is one of starvation from nutrients and excess of empty calories. By eating the right natural foods as the basis of your diet, you will be well on your way to achieving the right weight and the health you deserve. Ancient humans, after the control of fire, were also eating both raw and cooked foods intermittently.

6. Consume Foods That Will Minimize Burden of the Body

Foods that burden your body are unnatural foods filled with chemical products that increase their taste and color unnaturally. They weigh down the body and require it to spend energy on the elimination of such chemicals rather than focusing on achieving and maintaining health. Undigested foods rotting in our digestive system also form an extreme burden on our bodies. Due to the increased overload of waste and unnatural products in our body from eating

Chapter 13 - So, What Should We Eat... and Why?

unnatural foods, eating foods in excess or eating indigestible food molecules, the immune system becomes overloaded and is less able to control cell growth and cell health. This often leads unwanted diseases to get out of control, such as cancer, that should have been recognized by our immune system and eliminated from the body in its early stages.

Often, our body surrounds toxic substances with a fat layer or a fluid layer in order to isolate these toxins from other tissues. This makes removal of fat tissue and excess fluids sometimes especially difficult.

Foods that burden the body include:

1. Foods with unnatural colorings which contain E numbers from E100–E199 (colors).
2. Foods with unnatural preservatives which contain E numbers from E220–E228, E280–E283 (preservatives).
3. Foods with synthetic antioxidant E319.
4. Foods with hydrolyzed vegetable protein.
5. Foods with added flavorings which contain E numbers from E600–E699 (flavor enhancers).
6. High salt foods impair electrolytic balance. Foods containing more than 1.5 g of salt per 100 g are considered to be high in salt. Salt becomes a burden to health only when consumed in excess. But salt products such as monosodium glutamate (MSG) found in salty foods and soup mixes, is toxic to our brain cells and may even cause neuron cell death by causing over excitation of these cells.
7. Protein rich foods that are also rich sodium nitrates which contain E numbers from E249–E252. When fried, these foods form nitrosamines which are carcinogenic. These foods include cured meats, cooked bacon, some cheeses, nonfat dry milk, hot dogs, and other cooked processed meat products. [508]
8. Too much alcohol is also a burden to the body. I am not suggesting that a glass of wine or an occasional beer are a burden on a person's health, but when taken in excess, alcohol damages

Chapter 13 - So, What Should We Eat... and Why?

the liver. Regularly drinking over 1.5 pints of beer or cider, one glass of wine (250 ml), or 3-4 shots of spirits per day for men, and for women 1 pint of beer or cider, one glass of wine (175 ml), or 2-3 shots of spirit per day, can increase your risk of developing liver disease and cause irreparable damage to this very important organ. Alcohol damages intestinal walls letting toxins from the gut bacteria get into the liver. These toxins also lead to inflammation and scarring. In good health, the liver helps the body to get rid of waste products and plays a vital role in fighting infections, particularly in the bowel. [509] The liver turns glucose into fat which it sends round the body to store for use when we need it. Also, the liver, when it is burdened with toxins, will create more fatty tissues to store the toxins instead of ridding them through other ways. Unfortunately when the liver gets damaged, you won't know it until a serious health situation develops such as "fatty liver." [510] If you stop drinking alcohol on a regular basis for only two weeks and don't exceed the guidelines above, as well as reducing the chemical toxins from your diet, the liver will start shedding excess fat. On the other hand, if you choose not to change your drinking or dietary patterns, fatty liver will lead to chronic liver disease and with time causing loss of liver function.

9. Research shows that chewing gum and dietary food products and drinks containing artificial sweeteners increase appetite and leave you with a feeling of hunger just 20 minutes after their consumption. Foods with a high aspartame concentration have a time-dependent, biphasic effect on appetite, producing a transient decrease followed by a sustained increase in hunger. [511] These stimulants have a very negative effect on your weight loss attempts as well as on our health. In fact, epidemiological studies support the association between artificially sweetened food and beverage consumption and weight gain in children. [512] Another effect of artificial sweeteners in chewing gum is that although they have no caloric value, when the body breaks them down, it forms formaldehyde and methanol which are very toxic substances for our bodies.

10. Excess oil in the diet burdens the body due to the sensitivity of oil to heat, light, and exposure to oxygen. When this happens, unsaturated fats oxidize which cause free radical damage to cells.
11. Genetically modified foods should be avoided. Governments and companies are trying to hide the truth about genetically modified (GMO) foods, and as long as they are making hefty profits from these foods and hold the power over global food sources in their hands, they will never allow for the truths about these foods to be made available to the public. The bottom line is that as of today, we do not have enough evidence whether these foods are destructive or not for our health. There are no long term studies on the effects these foods have on human health, and studies that do prove the unhealthy nature of these foods and their potential to lead to incurable and sometimes fatal neurological conditions (as was proven in the late 1980's through research by on genetically engineered L-Tryptophan supplements) are consistently hidden from the crowds. Nowadays, only by consuming organic produce can we avoid GMO foods. 94% of soy and over 80% of corn grown in the U.S. are genetically modified crops and without the knowledge and research about the after effects these foods have on our health, they are best avoided. (513)

Eating a healthy diet helps keep the immune system tough enough to maintain health, but there are also foods that support the elimination of toxins. The following foods help *remove* toxins from the body and support a healthy liver: Apples, artichokes, pineapples, lemons, parsley, cabbage, beetroot, garlic, ginger, seaweed, and green tea all have detoxifying potential. Also incorporating regular exercise into your daily regime is beneficial for reducing the burden of toxins on our bodies and reduce the threat of a fatty liver on our health.

7. Consume Foods Rich in Nutrients

Nutrients we consume from our foods have many important functions in our body. No single food provides all of the nutrients we need to be healthy. The key lies in varying our diet with different

Chapter 13 - So, What Should We Eat... and Why?

healthy food sources. The larger our dietary diversity, the better our chances of getting all of our necessary nutrients through our diet.

Below are the six nutrients we get from our foods and suggestions on how to get the most nutrients from the foods you consume:

(1) **Vitamins** help to regulate chemical reactions in the body. There are thirteen vitamins, including vitamin A, the eight B vitamins, C, D, E, and K. Because most vitamins cannot be made in the body, we must obtain them through the diet. The most vitamin rich foods are fruits.

(2) **Minerals** are involved in innumerable body functions including bone structure, blood structure, muscle contraction, waste removal, cell to cell signaling, and so much more. The most mineral dense foods are vegetables. Vegetables are not only nutrient dense, but they are also calorie meagre, so you *can* and *should* eat them in abundance. Eating more vegetables and fruits can help you reduce the risk of heart disease and stroke by up to 30%. [514] A diet rich in vegetables and fruits has been proven to prevent certain types of cancer, help control blood pressure, avoid diverticulitis and other bowel diseases, and to protect against cataract and macular degeneration, two common forms of vision loss. [515, 516, 517, 518, 519, 520, 521, 522, 523, 524] The latest dietary guidelines, published every five years since 1980 by the Department of Health and Human Services (HHS) and the Department of Agriculture (USDA), recommends five to thirteen servings of fruits and vegetables a day (2½ to 6½ cups per day), depending on one's caloric intake. [525] For example, a person who needs 2,000 calories a day to maintain optimum weight and health, is recommended to consume nine servings, or 4½ cups of fruit and vegetables a day. (Two cups of fruit and 2½ cups of vegetables.)

(3) **Water** is another vital nutrient for good health. Most of our body weight (60-70%) is made up of water. Water helps control our body temperature, it carries nutrients and waste products from our cells, and is needed for our cells to function. Water is found in abundance in both fruit and vegetables. Gorillas rarely drink water

Chapter 13 - So, What Should We Eat... and Why?

since the foods they consume are so rich in water. Although we do need to drink more since we sweat more due to our comparatively hairless bodies, the best way to hydrate our body is by drinking plain water. Water is the most natural way to hydrate our body and it comes without the excess calories we get from sodas. Available data indicates a clear and consistent association between soft drink consumption and increased energy intake/calorie intake. Soft drinks have such a substantial impact on total energy intake it is therefore wise to recommend a decrease in their consumption. Soft drinks offer much energy with little accompanying nutrition. In fact, soft drinks displace other nutrients, especially magnesium, potassium, and calcium and are linked to several key health conditions such as diabetes. [526] and osteoporosis.

(4) **Carbohydrates** can be grouped into two categories: simple and complex carbohydrates. Simple carbohydrates are sugars or simple starches, and complex carbohydrates consist of starch and dietary fiber. Carbohydrates provide us with energy that is used mainly to fuel muscles and the brain, and therefore most of our daily caloric intake should come from healthy complex carbohydrates. Healthy sources of complex carbohydrates include whole grain products such as wholegrain breads, whole grain cereals, whole grain pastas, and whole grain types of rice as well as fruits and vegetables.

(5) **Protein** from food is broken down into amino acids by our digestive system which is then used for building and repairing body tissues and for making hormones. Protein intake is also important for a healthy immune system. Protein is also a source of calories and can be used for energy if not enough carbohydrates are available in the diet due to irregular eating patterns, intensive exercise, or extreme dieting. Healthy sources of protein include foods which can be consumed in abundance such as all types of beans, lentils, peas, nuts, and seeds. Grass fed or naturally raised animal meats and fish may also be consumed although only on rare occasions during the week.

(6) **Fat** is another nutrient we get from food which plays an important role in our health. Fat maintains healthy skin and hair, cushions our inner vital organs, provides insulation from heat and

cold, and is necessary for the production and absorption of certain vitamins and hormones. Our diet should include more unsaturated fats. Animal-based foods such as meats and milk products are higher in saturated fat whereas most vegetable sources are higher in unsaturated fat. Each gram of fat provides more than twice the amount of calories per gram of carbohydrates or proteins consumed. Healthy vegan sources of fat include seeds, nuts, and avocados. Fruits are also rich in fatty acids.

8. Consume Foods Rich in Fiber to Increase Digestion and Waste/Toxin Removal Rate

Fiber is important for health even though it is not really digested. Fiber is found in natural food sources and is lacking in processed foods. In the foods we consume, we can find two types of fiber: soluble and insoluble fiber.

Soluble fiber is found in fruits, nuts, legumes, seeds, and whole grains. Soluble fiber turns into a gel like substance which slows its digestion thereby lowering cholesterol and helps control blood sugar levels while providing very little energy in the form of calories. Insoluble fiber is found in vegetables, nuts, the skin of fruits, and also in whole grains. This type of fiber does not provide any calories and helps remove toxins and waste products from our body as well as prevent constipation or diverticulitis. [527] Insoluble fiber has also been shown to reduce the risk for developing colon cancer. [528, 529] High-fiber foods take longer to digest, keeping you satisfied for longer.

Table 7: *The Guerrilla Diet and Lifestyle Program Recommended* **Foods Rich in Fiber**

Food Source	Fiber (grams per cup)
Split Peas	16

Food Source	Fiber (grams per cup)
Lentils	15.5
Beans	15
Artichoke	10
Peas	9
Berries	8
Avocado	7
Whole Wheat Grains Including Oats	4.5 - 6.5
Chia and Flax Seeds	5.5

9. Consume Foods Low in Animal Protein

As I have stated in depth in Chapters 6 and 7, in order to avoid most modern day ailments, it is best to stick to a mostly vegan based, natural, whole food diet with meat consumption occurring on rare occasions weekly. If you decide to consume meat, your intake should be no more than 300 gm (11 oz.) a week, and of this amount, none, or as little as possible, should be from processed meats. Red meat should form no more then half to two-thirds of this weekly recommended amount (150-200 gm (5-7 oz.). These recommendations are very similar to the recommendations of the American Institute of Cancer Research on animal protein consumption. [530] If you choose to include eggs in your diet, go for the organic, free range eggs as they will be nutritionally healthier than eggs which come from chickens living in crowded enclosures, as they receive little to no antibiotics or hormones given in their feeds. An egg is equal to 50 grams (1.8 oz) of animal protein, so if you are vegetarian and choose to exclude dairy products, you may eat up to 6 eggs per week. If you do choose this option, the healthiest form of egg consumption is to boil them.

However, remember this: consuming animal protein is always a choice. There is no real need for much animal protein in your diet since we have so many tasty, naturally protein and fat rich vegan foods that give you none of the harmful effects of excess saturated, polyunsaturated fatty acids that is found in animal protein.

In order to reduce cravings for animal products, make sure you consume enough fat rich seeds and nuts in your diet.

10. Consume Foods Rich in Fatty Acid Precursors

The subject of fatty acid intake has been covered in depth in Chapter 4 under the heading "Gorilla and Human Omega-3 and Omega-6 Fatty Acid Requirements," and in Chapter 6 under the heading "Fish Consumption: The Facts." To summarize: we do not need to consume animal or fish products in order to get our omega-3 polyunsaturated essential fatty acids in sufficient quantities in our diet. The more of these foods we consume, the higher our risk of suffering from common Western world diseases. In fact fish produces these fats only once they feed on plants that produce omega-3 fatty acids. The omega 3 in fish oils is actually produced from plant-based products.

The healthiest omega-3 fatty acid rich foods include flax seeds, walnuts, chia seeds, beans, tofu and squash, as well as kale, spinach and algae. From these foods we can convert the precise quantity of omega-3 fatty acids that our body requires and no more.

11. Consume Foods That Prevent Calcium Loss

Calcium plays an important role in our health and is one of the most important minerals for the human body. Calcium helps form and maintain healthy teeth and bones. It also plays an important role in blood clotting, sending and receiving nerve signals, muscle contraction, the release of hormones and other chemicals, as

Chapter 13 - So, What Should We Eat... and Why?

well as in the maintenance of a normal heart rhythm. Insufficient levels of calcium in the diet will lead the body to remove calcium from bone tissue in order to ensure normal cell function. This can lead to weakened bones and eventually to osteoporosis.

A number of dietary factors affect calcium loss from the body. In order to reduce calcium loss from the body we must reduce the foods that increase calcium loss.

Foods that increase calcium loss include:

(1) Foods high in protein (over 15%) increase calcium loss through the urine. [531]
(2) Proteins from animal sources, especially processed animal products, are much more likely to cause calcium loss than protein naturally occurring in plant foods.
(3) Foods rich in sodium also increase calcium loss in the urine.
(4) Caffeine increases the rate at which calcium is lost through the urine.
(5) Smoking also increases the loss of calcium from the body. [532]

The best vegan sources of calcium are included in the following chart. (DV = Daily Recommended Values.)

Table 8: Foods Rich In Calcium Recommended by ***The Guerrilla Diet and Lifestyle Program***		
Food	Amount	Calcium (mg)
Sprouted sesame paste	2 Tbsp.	390 (40% DV)
Collard greens, cooked	1 cup	357 (36% DV)
Turnip greens, cooked	1 cup	249 (25% DV)
Tofu, processed with nigari*	4 ounces	130-400 (13-41% DV)
Tempeh	1 cup	184 (19% DV)

Chapter 13 - So, What Should We Eat... and Why?

Table 8: Foods Rich In Calcium Recommended by **The Guerrilla Diet and Lifestyle Program**

Kale, cooked	1 cup	179 (18.5% DV)
Soybeans, cooked	1 cup	175 (18% DV)
Bok choy, cooked	1 cup	158 (16% DV)
Mustard greens, cooked	1 cup	152 (15.5% DV)
Okra, cooked	1 cup	135 (14% DV)
Tahini	2 Tbsp.	128 (13% DV)
Navy beans, cooked	1 cup	126 (13% DV)
Almond butter	2 Tbsp.	111 (11.5% DV)
Almonds, whole	1/4 cup	94 (9.5% DV)
Broccoli, cooked	1 cup	62 (6.5% DV)

12. Consume Foods Rich in Both Calcium and Magnesium

Magnesium is an extremely important in the maintenance of good health. Magnesium is a critical co-factor in more than 300 enzymatic reactions in the human body. Magnesium is involved in energy production, oxygen uptake, central nervous system function, electrolyte balance, glucose metabolism and muscle activity, including the heart muscle. Magnesium is also an essential element in the construction of cell membranes and vitally important to the electrolyte balance of cells. When magnesium levels begin to drop, cells suffer from low energy production levels, electrolyte balance is disrupted, and the functional membrane system begins to fail leading to calcium and sodium fluctuating in and out of cells.

Due to the importance of calcium and magnesium in human health, it is wise to consume natural foods rich in these important minerals. Leafy greens are rich in both calcium and magnesium. However, some contain oxalic acid which can be found in spinach, rhubarb, chard, and beet greens. Oxalic acid binds with the calcium in these foods and reduces its absorption, but calcium in other green vegetables is well absorbed. [533, 534] Dietary fiber has little effect on calcium absorption. Higher levels of calcium and magnesium rich foods are especially important for post-menopausal women.

The best vegan sources of magnesium are included in the following chart:

Table 9: Magnesium Content in Foods Recommended by *The Guerrilla Diet and Lifestyle Program*

Food	Amount	Magnesium (mg)
Pumpkin Seeds	1/2 cup (113g)	606 (152% DV)
Brazil Nuts	1/2 cup (113g)	424 (106% DV)
Sesame Seeds	1/2 cup (113g)	396 (99% DV)
Almonds	1/2 cup (113g)	305 (77% DV)
Dark Leafy Greens (Raw Spinach)	1 cup cooked (180g)	157 (39% DV)
Soy Beans	1 cup cooked (172g)	148 (37% DV)
Brown Rice	1 cup cooked (195g)	86 (21% DV)
Chard	100 g cooked	86 (22% DV)
White Beans	100 g cooked	74 (19% DV)
Avocado	1 Avocado (200 g)	58 (15% DV)

Chapter 13 - So, What Should We Eat... and Why?

13. Consume Foods Rich in Methyl Donors

Foods rich in B vitamins act as methyl donors causing methyl groups to attach more frequently to specific genes thereby altering their expression, without altering the genomic structure of DNA. [535] In this manner, the methyl donors counteract detrimental effects induced by environmental toxins by influencing the epigenome in a positive way. [536] It is important to consume the foods in table 10 in abundance to ensure health and easy weight loss, and to reduce the tendency for obesity and diabetes.

Table 10: Foods Rich In Methyl Donors Recommended by *The Guerrilla Diet and Lifestyle Program*			
Food	Amount	B Vitamin	Content
Collard Greens	1 cup	Choline	73 mg (17% DV)
Broccoli	1 cup	Choline	55 mg (15% DV)
Swiss Chard	1 cup	Choline	50 mg (12% DV)
Cauliflower	1 cup	Choline	48 mg (11% DV)
Asparagus	1 cup	Choline	47 mg (11% DV)
Quinoa	1 cup	Betaine	630 mg (no DV)
Spinach	1 cup	Betaine	577 mg (no DV)
Lentils	1 cup	Folic acid	358 mcg (90% DV)

Table 10: Foods Rich In Methyl Donors Recommended by *The Guerrilla Diet and Lifestyle Program*

Food	Amount	B Vitamin	Content
Spinach	1 cup	Folic acid	263 mcg (66% DV)
Turnip Greens	1 cup	Folic acid	170 mcg (42% DV)
Broccoli	1 cup	Folic acid	168 mcg (42% DV)
Beets	1 cup	Folic acid	136 mcg (34% DV)
Romaine Lettuce	2 cups	Folic acid	128 mcg (32% DV)
Bok Choy	1 cup	Folic acid	70 mcg (17% DV)
Cauliflower	1 cup	Folic acid	55 mcg (14% DV)
Parsley	1/2 cup	Folic acid	46 mcg (12% DV)
Pinto Beans	1 cup	Folic acid	294 mcg (74% DV)
Garbanzo Beans	1 cup	Folic acid	282 mcg (71% DV)
Black Beans	1 cup	Folic acid	256 mcg (64% DV)
Navy Beans	1 cup	Folic acid	255 mcg (64% DV)

Chapter 13 - So, What Should We Eat... and Why?

Table 10: Foods Rich In Methyl Donors Recommended by ***The Guerrilla Diet and Lifestyle Program***			
Food	Amount	B Vitamin	Content
Kidney Beans	1 cup	Folic acid	230 mcg (58% DV)
Papaya	1 medium	Folic acid	102 mcg (26 % DV)
Brussels Sprouts	1 cup	Folic acid	94 mcg (23% DV)
Peas	1 cup	Folic acid	87 mcg (22% DV)

14. Consume Foods Rich in Prebiotics

Scientists are now beginning to understand that when taking the numbers into consideration, we are only about 30% human! The rest of us is made up of microorganisms, mainly bacteria. We have about 40 trillion cells in our body and about 20-30,000 human protein-coding genes, whereas we have about 100 trillion **microorganisms** living in our tissues and fluids (about three times the amount of cells we have). Together these microorganisms are called our microbiome. Our microbiome includes a whole range of microorganisms estimated from 700-1000 different species with about 3 million microbial genes! They outnumber our genes by an estimated 10-fold!

The microbes in our bodies weigh about 2-3 kilograms (5.5 lbs). The microorganisms that colonize our body compete with our cells for nutritional resources which we get from our diet.

We have a very close relationship with these microbes. Some microbes help us in many ways, and yet other microbes are harmful to us through the metabolites they produce. One thing is for sure; our microbiome affects us in ways we are only beginning to understand.

Chapter 13 - So, What Should We Eat... and Why?

Each and every one of us has our own unique and special microbiome template. Our microbiome functions to ensure proper digestive functioning of our foods, especially foods that the stomach and small intestine have not been able to digest. Microbiome also helps with the production of some vitamins (B12 and K) and plays an important function in our immune system. Microbiome begins colonizing our intestine right after birth and evolves as we grow as a result of different environmental influences and our diet. Microbiome adapts to changes in our diet and environment although in extreme cases of neglect, nutritional deficiencies, stress, and a very sedentary lifestyle, steer to a loss of balance in gut microbiome leading the harmful bacteria to flourish while beneficial bacteria decline. This loss of balance is linked to health problems such as obesity, bowel disorders, inflammatory bowel disease, certain cancers, allergies and diabetes.

But How Do These Small One-Cell Microbes Influence Our Health So Dramatically?

It's correct that they ARE small, but in large numbers, they markedly influence our health, in fact, microbes have systems in place to determine whether they are in minority or in majority at all times.

The microbes invade our body and wait until they are in sufficient numbers, and when they reach high enough numbers, they turn on group behaviors that either support or harm our health. They also have a mechanism in place by which they can "count" our cells, so they always know who is the majority and who is in the minority. Through this information, they decide which behaviors to take part in as a group.

Our microbiome directly influences our health and weight.

Microbes in our gut can manipulate our brain, our eating behaviors, and our mood to support their needs. When they live in our body, they rely on the foods we eat to support their needs, and when the microbes are in sufficient numbers, be they healthy or

Chapter 13 - So, What Should We Eat... and Why?

unhealthy bacteria, they will influence our eating patterns depending on their needs.

Some bacteria feed on sugar and simple carbohydrates, others prefer fiber and others feed on substances found only in meat and dairy. The population of microbes we support in our gut is therefore dependent on the foods we eat on a regular basis.

Gut bacteria support their own survival through two mechanisms:
1. The bacteria generate food cravings for foods that promote their survival or for foods that suppress their competitors survival
2. The bacteria induce unhappiness until we eat the foods that support their survival. They do this by producing toxins that influence our mood, change our taste receptors [537] to crave certain foods, and they are even capable of "hijacking" our vagus nerve, a long nerve that runs between the gut lining and our brain.

Evidence suggests [538] that the vagus nerve regulates eating behavior and body weight.

Certain bacteria stimulate vagus nerve activity which appears to drive excessive eating behavior [539] even when we are full.

Together these results suggest that microbes control our eating behaviors.

We now know that lean individuals, tend to have a wider variety of bacteria in their microbiome whereas overweight individuals have less diversity of their microbe population.

The more diverse the group of microbes we have in our gut, the more the bacteria compete with each other for space and nutrients, and this situation is better for us, because highly diverse populations of gut microbes expend more energy and resources in competition with each other, in comparison to a less diverse microbial population which becomes very powerful over us and can manipulate our eating behaviors more readily and with much more impact. Put simply, the larger the microbial community is, the more power it has to manipulate our dietary choices and influence unhealthy food consumption patterns and weight gain so the more diverse our microbial population is, the better our health.

Although early exposure is the key determinant of adult microbe population, we do have control over the composition of our gut microbiome through our diet, our lifestyle choices and our environment. An unhealthy diet, obesity, psychological stress, vitamin D deficiency, and pollution will influence our microbiome.

We can easily manipulate the composition of our gut bacteria with the following recommendations:

Prebiotic rich foods provide nourishment for the good bacteria which helps them to thrive and multiply. Prebiotics include Inulin, Xylo-oligosaccharides, Arabinogalactan, Fructo-oligosaccharides (FOS), Galacto-oligosaccharides (GOS). Prebiotics do not digest in the stomach or small intestine, and are accessible to the good bacteria once the food source reaches the large intestine. Prebiotics have been shown to prevent colorectal cancer. [620] Harmful microbes also affect the brain. The toxic metabolic by-products, and inflammatory molecules produced by the harmful bacteria in the gut adversely affects the brain.

Obesity has been linked to a harmful microbiome. In a study published in the journal *Diabetes* in 2007 [540] researchers identified that harmful bacteria produce toxins called lipopolysaccardies (LPS) which trigger inflammation as well as insulin resistance thereby promoting weight gain. Furthermore, gut microbes are thought to be key players in fat absorption and in the gain of more energy from the diet. [541] A diet rich in prebiotics leads to a reduction in the amount of fat and energy absorbed from food.

Prebiotics occur naturally in different plant-based foods. Consuming prebiotic rich foods will help create a beneficial gut microbiome to help ward off many modern day diseases. Prebiotic rich foods include: all types of onions, garlic, asparagus, Jerusalem artichokes, artichokes, chicory root, dandelion greens, whole grains, soybeans and other pods vegetables, beans, plums, bananas, and black grapes, raisins, as well as fresh honey, nuts, seeds.

Also, spend more time outside and open windows while in the house or office to help increase the diversity of your microbiome.

Chapter 13 - So, What Should We Eat... and Why?

But best of all [542] is to get out into nature at least once a week to do some kind of physical activity like a walk in nature so that you fill your body with healthy microbes from the air you breath. The airborne microbiome of the built environment is very different [543] from the microbiome in the outdoor nature environment.

I also recommend you reduce the use of antibiotics (use only when absolutely necessary). Broad spectrum antibiotics kill your microbiome and it may take months to rebuild again.

Also cut nonorganic meat, dairy and poultry products from your diet as much as possible. The animals are given antibiotics on a regular basis due to their confined living conditions and the easy spread of disease.

In general, lowering the amount of animal products you consume will help you maintain a healthier microbe population. Animal products encourage the growth of specific bacteria that are harmful to your health. Animal products increase the abundance of bile-tolerant microorganisms (*Alistipes*, *Bilophila* and *Bacteroides*) and decrease levels of Firmicutes that metabolize dietary plant polysaccharides. The amounts and activity of *Bilophila wadsworthia* on the animal-based diet support a link between dietary fat, bile acids and the outgrowth of microorganisms that may trigger inflammatory bowel disease. [544]

I also recommend that you allow yourself to get dirty from time to time, and the same goes for your kids. Constant washing, sanitizing and keeping the kids out of the dirt and sand will reduce their microbial diversity by not only killing bad bacteria, but also killing the good bacteria. We have always been in direct contact with dirt and our foods were taken directly from the ground. We need not be hysterical about a little dirt.

And lastly, if you have a choice of the method of giving birth to your children, choose natural childbirth through the birth canal as opposed to going for a caesarean birth. And opt to breastfeed your children at least up until solid foods are introduced to their diet at around 7 months. When newborns traverse the birth canal, they come into contact with microbes from their mother that help them to digest the milk. C-section babies skip this stage. Babies raised on formula milk face the disadvantage of not getting substances in breast milk that support the growth of beneficial microbes and limit the colonization of the gut with harmful ones. According to a recent Canadian study, babies drinking formula milk in the early months, have microbes in their gut that are not seen in breast-fed babies until solid foods are introduced. The presence of these microbes at an early age, before the gut and immune system are mature, may be one reason [545] these babies are more susceptible to allergies, asthma, eczema and celiac disease, as well as obesity.

15. Get Sufficient Vitamin D

An estimated 1 billion people from all ethnicities and age groups are vitamin D deficient in the world today. [546, 547, 548]

Previously, Vitamin D the essential fat-soluble, hormone-like vitamin was known to be used by the body for the proper absorption of calcium, bone development and maintenance of healthy bones and teeth and adequate phosphorus uptake.

We previously knew that vitamin D deficiency was involved in osteomalacia (a condition of weakened muscles and bones) and rickets (a disease in which bones fail to develop properly), due to the high numbers of rickets cases in the early 1900's, Vitamin D was added to processed foods to prevent deficiency.

Nowadays vitamin D research has come a long way due to the cheap testing available allowing scientists to take a deeper look at this vitamin and its effects on our health.

Vitamin D: Health Benefits:

We now know that Vitamin D is not only involved in bone and teeth health but also involved in:

Cell growth, proper neuromuscular functioning, proper immune function, proper brain function, and protects against many diseases and conditions including cancer, type 1 diabetes, multiple sclerosis, leukemia, and is also involved in weight loss.

Vitamin D and weight loss:

Chapter 13 - So, What Should We Eat... and Why?

A study to investigate the relationship between Vitamin D and measures of body size, composition, metabolism, and physical fitness in a young physically active population [549] revealed a significant negative relationship between BMI levels and serum levels of Vitamin D. The researchers also noted a positive correlation between cardiovascular fitness and Vitamin D3 levels.

A population-based prospective study in Rotterdam [550] with the objective to investigate the association between vitamin D status and body composition in the elderly, showed that low vitamin D concentrations are associated with a higher fat mass percentage in people over the age of 55 years. Furthermore, Vitamin D status was found to be positively associated [551] with lean body mass (LBM).

Researchers at the University of Minnesota [552] found that Vitamin D levels in the body at the start of a low-calorie diet predict weight loss success. Additionally, higher baseline vitamin D levels predicted greater loss of abdominal fat.

We now know that Vitamin D deficiency affects almost every organ and function of our body. But how is this possible?

The reason comes from two facts:

1. Vitamin D is not a vitamin. Vitamins are defined as an essential nutrients that the body cannot produce and must be acquired from our diet. Vitamin D is actually a hormone because it regulates body physiology and our bodies are capable of producing our own vitamin D through the action of sunlight on the skin. We never receive the vitamin itself, but a precursor to the vitamin that goes through a process in the liver and kidneys to produce the vitamin for use by the body. We are actually getting the vitamin D precursor from our diet or the sunlight, and then it is converted into vitamin D3, the active form in our kidneys.

2. Vitamin D influences the expression of genes. [553] It is needed for all cell renewal and protein transcription due to its role in allowing access to the DNA of the cell and allowing the cells to get the information needed for protein production. Therefore, we have Vitamin D receptors in almost all cells of our body including bone

cells, white blood cells, muscle cells, heart tissue cells, brain cells, endocrine glands, prostate gland, etc.

For these reasons, when we have vitamin D deficiency, it wreaks havoc on the whole body. For example, deficiency in vitamin D is now known to lead to: A weakened immune system, [554] increased cancer risk, [555] poor hair and nail growth, cognitive impairment and loss of balance in older adults, increased risk of death from heart disease, increased risk of prostate cancer, [556] and leukemia, inadequate insulin levels and decreased lung function.

But why are we deficient in vitamin D?

Vitamin D is imperative to our health and throughout our history, living on the Savannah grasslands of Africa for over 2 million years until some groups migrated out of Africa 60,000 years ago, we were receiving plenty of sunlight without any risk of deficiency from this nutrient.

But nowadays, things are different.

1. We spend much of our days in offices. We arrive early in the morning and leave after dark never to see enough of the healthy UVB rays from sunlight that convert cholesterol on our skin into calciol (vitamin D3). Vitamin D3 moves to the liver where it is converted into calcidiol (25-hydroxyvitamin D3). When vitamin D is needed, it is moved into the kidneys and transformed into the active form of vitamin D, called calcitriol (1,25-hydroxyvitamin D3). The conversion to calcitriol is regulated by its own concentration, parathyroid hormone, and serum levels of calcium and phosphate.

2. The modern use of statins and other medications or supplements that inhibit cholesterol synthesis, liver function or kidney function impair the synthesis of vitamin D and lead to its deficiency.

3. Furthermore, since the early 1950's, the food industry supplemented processed foods with vitamin D so that people wouldn't suffer from rickets, but nowadays, people are becoming wiser consumers and fewer people are consuming processed foods, so we see vitamin deficiency spring up again.

4. But not only that, even when we go on holiday to warm countries, we've become so scared of the sun that we use powerful

Chapter 13 - So, What Should We Eat... and Why?

sunscreens which reflect the healthy UVB radiation away. We still should use sunscreen because the ozone layer isn't whole as it was in the days before the industrial revolution, but I suggest only using sunscreen after getting sufficient sunlight to make vitamin D as presented in Table 12.

5. It is not easy to get vitamin D from foods, only very few foods have the provitamin available.

6. UVB radiation is most active between 11 in the morning and three in the afternoon in places and times where available. During the other hours, UVA radiation is more prominent and doesn't supply us with vitamin D. However, if you live on a longitude line above 35°, during the winter months you will not have any UVB radiation. This radiation doesn't reach the northern hemisphere in winter.

How can you know whether you are Vitamin D deficient or not?

A simple blood test can determine your vitamin levels, and levels below 40 ng/mL are considered a deficiency. The optimal range being 40-60 ng/mL.

You probably are deficient in Vitamin D if any of these apply to you:

1. You have a dark skin tone

Darker skinned populations that are living at high latitude lines are at greater risk for vitamin D deficiency because darker skins need more sun exposure to produce the same amount of vitamin D as pale skin does. Skin pigmentation acts as a natural sunscreen. The darker you are, the more pigment you have, and the more pigment you have, the more time you'll need to spend in the sun to make adequate amounts of vitamin D.

2. You feel depressed

The feel-good hormone serotonin is raised with exposure to sunlight and decreases with little sun exposure. In 2006, a study examined the effects of vitamin D on the mental health of 80 elderly patients and found those deficient in vitamin D were eleven times

more prone to depression than those who had sufficient vitamin D through supplementation.
3. You're aged 60 +
When you age, your skin makes less vitamin D in response to UVB exposure. Your liver and kidneys may not be in their best condition, and the kidneys may not be converting vitamin D into the active D3 form efficiently.
4. You suffer from bone pain
According to Dr. Michael F. Holick, an American endocrinologist specializing in the field of vitamin D for over 40 years states that people who see their doctor for aches and pains, especially in combination with fatigue, may be misdiagnosed as having fibromyalgia or chronic fatigue syndrome when they actually have a vitamin D deficiency. He explains: "What's happening is that the vitamin D deficiency causes a defect in putting calcium into the collagen matrix into your skeleton. As a result, you have throbbing, aching bone pain."
5. Being overweight or having a high muscle mass
People who are overweight or obese (or have a higher muscle mass) have higher needs for Vitamin D because body fat collects the vitamin D. Being overweight or obese, increases vitamin D requirements, and the same goes for weight lifters and body builders with increased muscle mass.

So how do we ensure we get enough of this vital nutrient?
1. Sunlight
Get some sunlight before applying sunscreen. But how much is enough? Depending on the number of UVB rays available. Today any weather app also shows you the UV index for your location, and you can use it to determine how much sunlight you need to get for optimal vitamin D intake in the following table:

Vitamin D, Skin Type and Exposure Recommendations

Chapter 13 - So, What Should We Eat... and Why?

Skin Type	UV Index 0-2	UV Index 3-5	UV Index 6-7	UV Index 8-10	UV Index 11+
Always burns/ Doesn't tan	None	10-15 min	5-10 min	2-8 min	1-5 min
Easily burns/ Rarely tans	None	10-20 min	10-15 min	5-8 min	2-8 min
Sometime burns/ Slowly tans	None	20-30 min	15-20 min	10-15 min	5-10 min
Rarely burns/ Rapidly tans	None	30-40 min	20-30 min	15-20 min	10-15 min
Never Burns/ Always dark	None	40-60 min	30-40 min	20-30 min	15-20 min

When sunlight reaches our skin, it is also involved in the production of endorphins which make us feel good and feel happier. Sunlight exposure in moderation has even been shown to reduce the risk of skin cancer.Expose your skin to sunlight in moderation, and you will be healthier and happier. Note that Vitamin D has a half-life of only two weeks, meaning that stores can run low after two weeks, especially during the winter.

2. Food

Previously we thought that the only natural foods that contain sufficient vitamin D were oily fish, and mushrooms. Now we know that also many types of meat provide vitamin D. If we live above 35 longitude line and we don't eat or meat we may feel depressed especially during winter months. The reason is not that we lack meat but rather that vitamin D levels are low. Oily fish such as Mackerel provide 100% of our daily recommended need of Vitamin D per 3 oz portion, smoked Salmon provides 90% of our daily recommended need of Vitamin D per 3 oz portion, Canned Trout provides 94% of our daily recommended requirement of Vitamin D per 3 oz portion. Mushrooms may be a great source of natural vitamin D when the mushrooms are exposed to sunlight before their consumption. This action increases their vitamin D levels. So if mushrooms are placed outside in the suns UVB rays before adding them to your food, you will get sufficient vitamin D if you eat them daily. For example, Maitake mushrooms provide 131% of our daily recommended need of Vitamin D per cup; Portobello mushrooms provide 74% of our daily recommended need of Vitamin D per cup, Morel mushrooms provide 23% of our daily recommended requirement of Vitamin D per cup.

Keep in mind, from the foods we eat, we get vitamin D in the form D2 (ergocalciferol), which is metabolized differently from D3 (cholecalciferol) and less efficient on a per mole basis.

3. UVB Narrowband Lamps

Similar to tanning beds, but not quite the same, they provide access to only the good UVB radiation without the skin burning and skin cancer causing waves. That's why they are called narrowband because they provide light radiation in a small light bandwidth (295-311 nanometers). These solve the problem for anyone living above the 35° latitude line during the long winter months deprived of the beneficial UVB radiation.

4. Supplementation

It is best to obtain some vitamin D through your diet and to concentrate on getting sufficient sunlight exposure. That being said, during the winter months, if you believe you lack vitamin D due to your location and your skin tone, I suggest you take Vitamin D supplements. The total recommended intake can vary from about 2000 IU to 4000 IU per day, [556] including what you get from your diet and sunlight. If you are using supplementation, go for about 2000 IU per day and ensure that the supplement you choose to buy has no more than two ingredients, (olive oil and vitamin D3). This conscious consumption will help prevent regular intake of different chemicals into your body. Furthermore, when you take vitamin D as a supplement, you're creating an increased demand for Vitamin K2. Your body will make more vitamin K2-dependent proteins that will move the calcium around the body. These have a lot of potential health benefits. But until the K2 comes in to activate those proteins, those benefits aren't realized. Therefore, when supplementing daily with Vitamin D, take vitamin K2 three times per week. Vitamins D and K2 work together to improve your heart health and strengthen your bones. Vitamin K2 is mainly found in specific animal foods and fermented foods, which most people don't eat much of. Vitamin K2 is also produced by gut bacteria in the large intestine, and there is some evidence that use of broad-spectrum antibiotics can contribute to K2 deficiency.

Vitamin D made from sunlight will last 2 to 3 times longer in the body than vitamin D taken as a supplement.

Note: Although rare, excess vitamin D can be reached with excess supplementation. Excessive supplementation will lead the body to absorb too much calcium, leading to increased risk of a heart attack as well as kidney stones. 20,000 IU is the toxicity level.

16. During The Day Consume Foods Regularly So As To Avoid Strong Feelings Of Hunger. During The Night Go On An Intermittent Fast Of 12 Hours.

Can you imagine that you just started a new diet that doesn't allow eating any carbohydrates, meaning no bread, no pasta, no rice, etc., and you are feeling very hungry? Then your friend comes along from the bakery with a bag of freshly baked croissants. She offers you one and since you feel like you're starving, what do you think you're going to do? Well, of course you're going to eat it because you're feeling hungry!

Willpower is not enough to overcome your survival mechanism which is stronger than anything else. We are programmed to survive, and to do this we need food, and when we are hungry any food will do. Without understanding this point and making sure that you are never hungry, you will not succeed at dieting and losing weight. And it is not only important to make sure that you're never hungry, it is also just as important to make sure that when you are hungry that you put in the proper foods into your body. So how do you do this?

Chapter 13 - So, What Should We Eat... and Why?

Remove all tempting sugar rich foods from all of your cupboards and your refrigerator. In fact, try to remove all of the unnatural processed foods from your kitchen. People don't really understand this concept, but none of the other steps that follow will matter if this one is not taken care of first. You see, when you do get hungry, you will tend to reach out to those foods that are easily accessible and consumed without needing almost any work on your behalf. Those foods most appealing to you will be stuck in front of your face if you leave them in your cupboards and fridge, and they will always test your willpower. We don't want this to happen, so remove the temptations. We want life to be easy, right?

The second step take is to make sure that you have good foods readily available to eat at all times to maintain a steady blood sugar level. For example, in the morning you can chop up some vegetable sticks and put them in a cup in the fridge to have ready for you to eat whenever you get hungry. The veggie sticks can be pepper sticks, carrots sticks, celery sticks, and so on. Have some cherry tomatoes washed and ready to eat as well as some fruit you especially like that you can carry with you to work, such as bananas, apples, or oranges. I also recommend having some nuts handy in a small box. These are great to calm you down when nervous and they also reduce the craving for meat and animal products. If you get really hungry and need something filling, you can also have a slice of healthy bread handy in a sandwich bag, topped with some sesame seed spread or another healthy spread option.

If you make sure that you are never really hungry and have foods available for you to eat when you do feel even the slightest urge to eat, then you will never feel starved and you will be able to have the sufficient willpower needed to say no when very appealing foods are presented to you.

Let's take an animal as an example. Can you imagine your pet cat saying no to any food that you give it when it is starving? Or your dog saying, "Oh, I don't know if this is healthy option for me. I won't have any of that!" when it's hungry? Of course not! But when they are full they won't be tempted by anything.

Chapter 13 - So, What Should We Eat... and Why?

Making sure that you will never be hungry is the easiest and the most cost-effective way to make sure that you will succeed at dieting and at achieving your health goals.

Now what if your friend was to come over and offer you a croissant when you had just eaten a few nuts and a healthy, nutrient rich sandwich just before she arrived. Would you be saying yes to her offer, or would you more likely say "No thank you. I'm full?"

Now although it is important to prevent hunger during the daytime, the benefits of fasting at night are just as advantageous.

Fasting as a method of healing has been around for many years. When I began alternative nutrition studies, in 1992, before I completed my university studies in nutrition, biochemistry and medical science, I learned from books written by Dr. Henry Lindlahr, author of the backbone texts of naturopathic medicine. It was then that I first learned of the power of fasting.

Over the years, much research has come out on this subject, and most scientists agree that intermittent fasting of about 12 hours has shown to have beneficial effects on various chronic diseases including rheumatic diseases, metabolic disease, ongoing pain, hypertension, chronic inflammatory diseases, atopic diseases, and even psychosomatic disorders [557].

Ancient humans living on the Savannah grasslands of Africa were fasting regularly from before the sun set, when they were getting organized for sleep, until after sunrise, when they would get up in search of food.

In Africa, where ancient humans resided, the dark hours of the night and twilight hours typically last for 12 hours all year round. Therefore, the fasting of 12-13 hours was their daily norm.

But how does in intermittent fasting lead to all of these benefits?

The body enters starvation mode about eight hours after the last meal is eaten, when the gut finishes absorbing the nutrients from the food consumed.

When eating regularly, dietary and body glucose, which is stored in the liver and muscles, is used as the primary source of

Chapter 13 - So, What Should We Eat... and Why?

energy. Our liver holds our reservoir of glucose in the form of glycogen. Fasting typically depletes liver glycogen, and fat becomes the next energy source for the body.

The breakdown of fatty tissue into free fatty acids produces ketone bodies which are used as an alternate energy source.

The brain relies on these ketone bodies which are produced in liver cells for energy consumption.

During prolonged fasting of more than twenty-four hours, the body starts breaking down protein (e.g. muscle tissue) for energy, and therefore intermittent fasting is recommended as opposed to prolonged fasting.

The fast I recommend lasts for 12-13 hours, from the last meal consumed at night to the first meal eaten in the day. Even if you finished your last meal at 10:30 PM, no problem, just eat your first meal (breakfast) no earlier then 10:30 AM, but also not much later then 11:30 AM.

This provides a gentle transition from using glucose as the primary source of energy to using fat, and back to using glucose. This cycle prevents the breakdown of muscle tissue for energy while helping in the process of weight loss. The depletion of glycogen from liver cells leads to the breakdown of fats resulting in a reduction in body fat.

But weight loss is just one of the benefits of intermittent fasting.

Although losing weight also helps reduce cholesterol levels, reduce blood pressure, helps control diabetes and reduces inflammation from active fatty tissue, fasting has other benefits.

Here are 9 more health benefits associated with intermittent fasting:

1. When doing regular fasts, your body will release more endorphins into the blood, making you feel happier and more alert. Brain function is optimized, and from an evolutionary standpoint, this implies that maintenance of high cognitive function when food is scarce is of utmost importance for survival.

Chapter 13 - So, What Should We Eat... and Why?

2. Ketone bodies protect cells from aging by the donating carbon sources which provide nourishment for cells while reducing cellular aging. [558]

3. Intermittent fasting also modifies peripheral energy metabolism. The brain communicates with all of the peripheral organs involved in energy metabolism and enhances parasympathetic activity, the body's unconscious actions involved in "rest-and-digest" or "feed and breed" [559] activities that occur while at rest. During fasting, this results in improved gut motility, reduced heart rate, and reduced blood pressure.

4. Intermittent fasting enhances insulin sensitivity of muscle and liver cells when eating reducing the risk for diabetes and metabolic syndrome.

5. Intermittent fasting also reduces levels of oxidative stress and inflammation throughout the body and brain. The reduction of inflammation in the brain has been shown in animal models to lead to fewer clinical symptoms of neurological disorders such as Alzheimer's disease, Parkinson's disease, Huntington's disease [560], as well as stroke [561] and epileptic seizures [562] in humans.

6. Intermittent fasting has also been shown to prolong the lives of rats. [563] In humans this effect occurs through the increase in human growth hormone with intermittent fasting, which maintains health, fitness and longevity, and promotes the increase in muscle mass while increasing fat loss.

7. Intermittent fasting has positive effects on diabetes. Hyperglycemia is improved, and insulin sensitivity is increased. [564]

8. Intermittent fasting has been shown to have positive effects on heart disease and to prevent or reverse multiple sclerosis. [565, 566]

9. We know that an impaired gut microbiome is an important factor in the pathogenesis of weight gain and other disorders. Intermittent fasting affects the gut microbiome by helping a healthy group of mucin-degrading microbes to thrive. [567]

Although there are many benefits to intermittent fasting, I do not recommend it to certain populations where it may have adverse effects including low weight children, the elderly or individuals with a BMI of 19 or less.

For Vascular Disease Patients

If you are suffering from some form of vascular disease including heart disease, or have suffered from a stroke or transient ischemic accident, you should reduce inflammatory promoting foods (see guideline 2 in this chapter), increase fiber rich foods (see guideline 8 in this chapter) and reduce fatty foods as much as possible from your diet, and this includes reducing even added olive oil on your salads to a minimum. This may seem very difficult to do at first, but foods can be cooked with little to no added fat, and if fat is to be used, try coconut butter instead, in very moderate amounts. Coconut butter melts easily in any pot or pan and only half a teaspoon is required for an excellent stir fry vegetable dish. The natural taste of foods begins to reappear once fat is reduced to a minimum because fats conceal their natural flavor. Use other condiments to flavor salads including balsamic vinegar, soy sauce, mustard, garlic, ginger, or just simply pour some sesame seed spread (tahini) on your food.

For Diabetes Patients

If you suffer from diabetes, it is important to take extra care and make sure that your food is balanced with your insulin or oral medications (if used), and your exercise program in order to help manage your blood glucose levels.

Foods need to be eaten on a regular basis, and foods high in dietary fiber are healthy options that keep blood sugar levels steady throughout the day. ***The Guerrilla Diet and Lifestyle Program*** is perfect for people with diabetes although it is wise to reduce the fruit percentage of the diet and exchange it for a more non-starchy vegetable options. By consuming fruits with their peel and not in the form of juices or shakes, you will help keep your blood glucose levels more stable.

Chapter 13 - So, What Should We Eat... and Why?

For Pregnant or Lactating Mothers and Females during Menstruation

During menstruation and pregnancy, emphasis should be placed on iron rich foods with a squeeze of lemon to support iron absorption.

The best vegan sources of iron are included in the following chart:

Table 11: Iron Rich Foods Recommended by ***The Guerrilla Diet and Lifestyle Program***		
Food	Amount	Iron (mg)
Pumpkin Seeds	1/2 cup (113g)	10 (55% DV)
Soy Beans	1 cup (180g)	8.8 (49% DV)
Cashews	1 cup (129g)	7.8 (43% DV)
White Beans	1 cup cooked (180g)	6.6 (37% DV)
Lentils	1 cup cooked (180g)	6.6 (37% DV)
Dark Leafy Greens	1 cup cooked (180g)	6.4 (36% DV)
Swiss Chard	1/2 cup (113g)	4 (22% DV)
Quinoa	1 cup (185g)	2.8 (15% DV)
Oatmeal	1 cup cooked (180g)	2.5 (12% DV)

During pregnancy, a small portion (up to 400 gm/13 oz. per week) of lean meat or fish is recommended in order to supply the very high iron and B12 needs, although for vegans, supplementation with B12 in the form of methylcobalamine and gentle iron is also a healthy option.

Chapter 13 - So, What Should We Eat... and Why?

Weight Lifters/Body Builders and Athletes

Weight lifters/body builders and athletes generally preform more physical activity than ancient humans did. Therefore, elite athletes may supplement their diets with up to 400 gm (13 oz.) of meat or fish a week, and as little as possible should be processed. (This includes canned tuna or salmon.) All other people may abstain from animal products altogether if so desired or may consume 300 gm (11 oz.) animal products per week.

Getting Your Children into Healthy Eating Patterns

Involve your children in your new way of life. Bring them along grocery shopping with you and explain to them your new food choices. Chances are they will start asking questions, and by answering them you will repeat what you have learned, strengthening your own learning process and the new habits within your own mind.

By showing them how you choose to buy nutritionally similar but not so beautiful and perfectly shaped fruit and vegetables, especially organic and in season foods, you are teaching them a valuable lesson for life.

Always have food handy to feed them if they become hungry. Should they start requesting fast food, ice cream or candy, understand that they are indicating to you that they are hungry. Answer them that this is fine by you after they have consumed the healthy food you currently have on hand. Explain to them that once they finish the healthy foods, you will provide them with a desert or treat, but give them boundaries as to which desert they can choose from, such as sorbets, soy based ice-cream, watermelon, etc.

In order to reduce your child's meat and dairy food consumption, make sure your children eat enough seeds and nuts. Since they are so easy to transport in a small box or bag, you can always have them handy. For younger children, nut or seed spreads on sandwiches are a great alternative, along with natural, sugar-free jams to help them enjoy the taste even more. Also, you may want to arrange a visit to a meat packing facility during school breaks or as a school trip. It is important for children and for yourself to understand what happens before these types of foods reach the table.

When baking cakes together with children, choose to replace any oils written in the recipe with coconut butter. Replace sugar with rice or date malt or maple syrup. Replace dairy products with almond paste or almond/soy/coconut milk. You may also use a quarter of a cup of organic non-GMO corn flour or flax seed flour mixed with water or any non-dairy milk instead of an egg in any recipe.

Grow a garden together with your children, even in pots placed on your porch or balcony, to teach them where their food comes from, how crops grow, and what needs to be done from seed to harvest. Bring them along to farmers markets, even if this is not the easiest chore to do with children.

Get them used to drinking water by bringing home a water dispenser or having mineral water delivered to your home regularly. Nowadays there is a whole range of water dispensers, including multi-temperature ones, that provide instant hot and cold water and even some that provide instant sparkling water. Give your children the task of filling up their glass BPA-free water bottles before they leave for school.

Lastly, take your children out into nature for a walk at least twice a week for a minimum time of twenty minutes each outing. This will be both beneficial to you and your children's health as well as creating strong family bonds.

Lifestyle Recommendations

Buy products with low environmental impact. Not only will these products be beneficial to the environment, they will be of immediate benefit for your own health by reducing your exposure to pollutants. Cleaning materials containing bleach include chlorine gases that are unnatural substances that are very toxic to inhale. These bleaches are also used to whiten cotton balls so prefer organic bleach free cotton balls and organic panty liners. Try to purchase natural cleaning materials. They are just as good as their chemical counterparts, but crucially healthier.

Chapter 13 - So, What Should We Eat... and Why?

Buy healthier pots and pans, drinking bottles, and food storage boxes without BPA, a recognized carcinogen. Try to use natural cosmetics, soaps, and shampoos. Use a natural contraceptive for birth control such as the Lady Comp. And lastly, double insulate your windows in order to reduce the excessive use of fossil fuels which further pollute our planet when heating/cooling your home.

By consuming the above mentioned foods and reducing consumption of non-local, processed, and unnatural foods, as well as animal products, while making sure that you always have food at hand and never get too hungry, you're putting yourself in a great position to succeed at adopting a healthy lifestyle and achieving easy and natural weight loss.

As well, by utilizing products that have a low environmental impact, you are not only supporting your own personal health and easily losing weight in the process, you are also playing a significant role in conserving the planet. By making these dietary and lifestyle choices you are reducing the amount of deforestation and reducing the pollution of soils, the air we breathe, and maintaining our supply of water.

You are supporting natural and organic farming which re-mineralizes the soil with natural rock dust fertilizers instead of chemical ones with their destructive effects on our environment. You are helping to reduce the amount of grains fed to animals instead of feeding those grains to people where poverty and malnutrition are of major concern.

This way of life also reduces conflict between people as there is sufficient land to feed the world's population... if handled with care.

It is time for us humans, supposedly the most intelligent species on the face of the earth, to stop the destruction of our planet for our own short term benefit. By consuming the natural foods as recommended above, we are evolving to a higher level of consciousness where we are not abusing the abundance we have on earth, but rather living as one with it. In this manner we will be ready to coexist in harmony with the plants, trees, and natural reserves we have on earth, and well as the planet we share with the animals. And

Chapter 13 - So, What Should We Eat... and Why?

also, just as importantly, we will learn to live in greater accord with each other.

Chapter 14

The Guerrilla Diet Shopping List

"The self is not something ready-made, but something in continuous formation through choice of action."

— John Dewey

In this chapter we shall go over the recommended foods on ***The Guerrilla Diet and Lifestyle Program.*** Consume the foods in the following lists daily in order to increase your health, longevity, and vitality, as well as help you to lose weight.

In this section we are not yet going into portion sizes. Here we are just examining which departments of the supermarket or farmers market you should be visiting.

Foods Recommended on The Guerrilla Diet:

Fruit
All fruits, either in their natural state or cooked, dehydrated or dried, but not juiced.

Vegetables
All vegetables – raw or cooked, but not juiced.
All root and starchy vegetables – cooked, baked, or mashed.
All mushrooms – raw or cooked.

Chapter 14 - The Guerrilla Diet Shopping List

Grains

All whole grains — raw or cooked. Try to vary your diet as much as possible on a weekly basis. Dietary diversity ensures you get the different nutrients available from different foods. Try to incorporate all types of grains including brown rice, wild rice, Indian red rice, buckwheat, millet, quinoa, spelt, kamut, amaranth, etc.

Fats

Coconut – raw or as butter or milk.

Cacao – powder or in the form of chocolate bars, 85% chocolate or darker.

Avocado – raw.

Nuts – raw or as butter or milk.

Seeds – raw or as butter or milk.

Olives – in brine. Also olive oil in very small quantities if desired, but not for cooking or baking.

Vegan Proteins

All local lentils.
Peas.
All local beans.

Animal Proteins

Up to 300 gm per week cooked, grilled, boiled, or oven baked. Organic, grass fed lean meat or free range chicken.

Fish – Atlantic mackerel, freshwater Coho salmon, wild-caught Pacific sardines, and Alaskan wild-caught salmon.

Organic, free range eggs, or pastured eggs from a local farmer.

Beverages

Water.
Sparkling water.
Coffee, freshly ground.
Tea – green or herbal.

Spices

All spices – fresh or dried.
All herbs.
Himalayan salt.
Seaweed.
Use unsweetened condiments (Balsamic/apple cider/wine vinegar, soy sauce, mustard, ketchup, tomato paste, relish).
Garlic.
Ginger.
Tahini.
Fermented, low salt condiments (Relish, sauerkraut).

Sweeteners

Stevia.
Honey (Raw unfiltered, local).

Chapter 15

Think and Grow Slim

"All that we are is a result of what we have thought"

— Buddha

For changing any lifestyle habit, new brain cell connections must be formed. To reprogram your mind so as to change your lifestyle choices and habits, you are going to need to build new brain and nervous system (neural) networks. In order to build new neural networks we need to focus our attention on the skill we want to improve and on the end process we wish to achieve with these new lifestyle changes. When we mentally attend to whatever we are learning, the brain can map the information on which we are focusing. How are new neural connections built to last so that our new lifestyle changes become lifelong habits? This is what we shall cover in this chapter.

Dr. Donald Hebb, a Canadian psychologist, published several important ideas in the field of neuroscience. One was known as the "Hebb synapse:" a theory explaining how neurons develop a relationship with one another. "When an axon of cell A is near enough to excite cell B and repeatedly or persistently takes part in firing it, some growth process or metabolic change takes place in one

Chapter 15 - Think and Grow Slim

or both cells such that A's efficiency, as one of the cells firing B is increased."

As Dr. Carla J. Shatz, an American neurobiologist and one of the pioneers of the basic principles of early brain development put it: "Neurons that fire together, wire together." When neurons are dedicated to a specific function, they wire together to create neural networks. [568] We now know that BDNF is one of the most active brain growth factors which acts on neurons and encourages their growth and differentiation into new neurons and synapses, helps support their survival, and helps create new neural networks. [569] BDNF is very important in helping us to form new behavioral patterns.

There are several ways to increase BDNF in the brain to help new lifestyle changes stick. As I described in Chapters 10 and 11, certain dietary guidelines, decreased caloric intake, physical exercise, repetition of thoughts and focusing ones attention will increase BDNF levels. [570, 571, 572, 573, 574]

In this chapter I shall point out the guidelines to help focus your attention, one of the basics to forming new and stronger neural networks.

It is important to mention that neural pathways are only maintained if you keep using them. This is both good and bad news. If you want to maintain a skill you must work at it and use it regularly. But the good news is, if you don't want to keep a non-beneficial neural network or behavior, then by not using it and not placing your attention on it, and by replacing it with an alternative neural network, you will support its disappearance (also called extinction) and support a new skill or behavior to take its place.

This is important news since you have the ability to change any lifestyle habit that is not useful, unwanted, and non-beneficial to you by focusing your attention elsewhere on what you *do* want to have in your life instead of what you don't want. By repeating some simple techniques you can change bad habits into good and beneficial ones, and maintain the new and better habits through maintenance of the new neural networks you have created once you begin ***The Guerrilla Diet and Lifestyle Program***.

Chapter 15 - Think and Grow Slim

This simple techniques involve focusing your attention on what you desire to have, be it weight loss or health, or really just about anything.

By maintaining attention towards one single visual picture you will actually change your brain structure by creating new and stronger neural networks to help you achieve your goals.

The Method

Reserve a daily time and place where you know that you will not be disturbed for at least fifteen minutes. Take a timer with you.

Set the timer for fifteen minutes then start it.

Close your eyes.

Take a slow, deep breath in.

Visualize a picture of yourself living with the end result of your goal, be it reaching a specific desired weight, radiating the health you want to have, doing a task you would love to do, or getting into the clothes you would love to see yourself wear. As you visualize this happening, announce repeatedly to your subconscious mind the goal that you are planning to reach. Remember that avoiding discomfort is the top priority of your reptilian brain, therefore your goal must provide you with great pleasure once achieved, and be attractive enough for you to overwhelm your reptilian brain programming to keep you on the right path towards achieving your goal.

Hold the visualization and the repeated thoughts of your goal for as long as you can until you are either distracted by another competing thought or the picture slowly fades away or changes form.

Stop the timer.

Restart the timer and do this again, but try to lengthen the time of the visualization process.

Do this technique repeatedly, at least once a day, preferably twice, and it will help you make your goal your reality because ***focus equals power***.

If you really find it hard to visualize the end result picture, don't worry. Instead, write down your goal and read it to yourself over and over during the day, every day. Read your weekly plan daily

Chapter 15 - Think and Grow Slim

as well to suggest that you are in full control of the situation. Feelings of control increase self-esteem and give you the energy, courage, and encouragement to go after the Fulfillment of your goals with persistence no matter what the current results seem to be.

Write your goal and weekly plan clearly on a sticky note in several copies and in wording that suggests that you have already achieved the goal. For example: "I weigh 60 kg.; I am radiating with good health; I look and feel great; I am so happy and grateful; I am successfully doing 'X' weekly goal." Hang these sticky notes wherever you can see them several times a day, including on your bathroom mirror so you see it first thing in the morning. Include them on the dashboard of your car and on your computer screen.

Focus your mind for a minute or two on the final outcome when you read your goal during the day.

You will undoubtedly reach your goal if you focus your attention on it and on the small steps needed to get you there. In the next chapter you will prepare a schedule of your weekly plans which will get you from where you are today to where you desire to be.

Chapter 16

The 12 Week Guerrilla Diet & Lifestyle Program

"You were born to win, but to be a winner, you must plan to win, prepare to win, and expect to win."

– Zig Ziglar

We need to have goals so that we know where we are going. If you don't know where you are going, you are like a car barreling down the highway without a driver at the wheel. You will certainly not reach the destination you desire if you do not have your hands firmly on the steering wheel and steer the car in the direction you want to proceed. This is the reason why goals and plans are so important. The weekly plan is there to help you create the small steps towards reaching your end goal. The steps are gradual and this type of change won't overwhelm you and trigger your reptilian brain to fight against your efforts. By following these weekly plans, slowly but surely you will be removing the negative lifestyle habits that perhaps have been giving you immediate or short- term gratification, but in the long run are leading to your self-destruction.

By using this gradual method, you are not only focused on your lifestyle habits that need changing, you are also focused on the

Chapter 16 - The 12 Week Guerrilla Diet & Lifestyle Program

action and not the result. Thus, fear from the unknown and fear of not reaching your end result, which is probably way out of your comfort zone, do not come into the equation. Fear is not felt and you are more in control of your destiny. In this gradual method, you can reach your goals in a more relaxed and controlled way.

The 12 weekly plans provide you with a weekly goal for you to focus on and conquer, and keep you on the right track to success.

Each of the twelve weeks you will focus on one goal specified in the list below . **Each week is built on the previous week and adds onto it, and does not replace it**.

Once you master the weekly goal, only then, proceeded to the next weeks destination. In this manner, you are placing your focus on lifestyle habit goals instead of focusing on your desired weight or health. These will come automatically as a result of changing your lifestyle habits, but your attention will be placed on where you want to be (on the positive outcome), rather than what you do not want in your life anymore and what you want to change (the negative current situation, the weight or health status you want to change). As I have explained, where you place your focus, neural networks will become stronger. If you place your focus on what you do not want to have in your life, you will just be strengthening this as a habit, and it will be more and more difficult to change this habit as time goes by. By focusing your attention on one goal a week you will find that you can achieve these goals and improve your health and lifestyle much easier than you thought was possible. Furthermore, when you begin achieving the little goals that will get you to where you want to be at the end of the program, your self-esteem will increase. You will believe in yourself and see that you are capable of achieving your desires. Once you gain control over yourself, you will find that you are able and can do anything you set your mind to do.

Begin each day by focusing your attention on how you will achieve your weekly goal. After the visualization technique, I recommend that you use your imagination to create strategies for you to achieve the weekly goal. This will plant the goal into your subconscious mind and create the basis for creating new neural networks that are more in tune with your health and weight loss goals.

The 12 Week Guerrilla Diet and Lifestyle Plan

You may, of course, change the order of these weekly plans to suit yourself although I have found that this particular order works best for most people.

WEEK 1

Choose to add more fresh or steamed green leafy and other vegetables to your existing diet.

This week have vegetables form one third to one half of each of your meals. By adding more vegetables to your diet, you will automatically reduce other, less nutrient dense foods from your diet and thus will be adding more vitamins and minerals making you feel healthier already. Compounds like sulforaphane in broccoli, diallylsulfide in garlic, and prebiotics found in onions, garlic, bananas, and artichokes, as well as selenium found in cabbage, green tea, soy, and Brazil nuts to name a few, promote a healthy gut microbiome and switch on anti-cancer genes to reduce the risk of heart disease, diabetes, obesity and certain cancers.

By adding vitamin/mineral/and fiber dense foods to your diet, you will feel fuller much sooner than if you were to be eating a diet rich in energy dense foods that are low in these nutrients.

Furthermore, by consuming vegetables that are also methyl donors, you are immediately influencing your DNA in a positive way and reducing any genetic tendency you may have to remain overweight and susceptible to disease in your life.

WEEK 2

This week reduce soft drinks to a minimum or preferably completely remove them from your diet, and focus on only

drinking pure water, sparkling (carbonated) water, natural caffeine-free teas or ground coffee this week.

Water is a major nutrient required to support our health. Water makes up about two-thirds of our body's weight. There is more water in the body than any other substance.

In Chapter 11 on physical activity, I mentioned the fact that humans have the ability to control their body temperature through sweating. We are, in fact, the species that sweats the most. Even on the coldest days we lose a minimum of 200 ml (1/2 pint) of water in the form of sweat. Therefore, unlike apes who rarely consume water, we do need to supplement our diets with water, and the water we get from foods is not enough to maintain optimum health. Drinking pure water helps maintain the balance of body fluids which are involved in digestive processes, absorption, the transport of nutrients to and from cells as well as toxin removal from the body, the formation of saliva, and maintenance of body temperature.

When drinking water, rather than any other beverage, you are satisfying your water needs without adding any energy in the form of calories to your diet, and without adding chemicals in the form of artificial sweeteners. Drinking water is also the healthier alternative because it does not change its osmolality and has no glycemic index unlike sugar and artificially sweetened beverages which directly affect blood sugar levels. Drinking water when hungry also makes you feel satiated.

Furthermore, water is a beneficial anti-aging nutrient allowing sufficient hydration which keeps the skin in good health and looking good. Also, any excess water consumed is always safely excreted by the kidneys.

Water removes waste products from our cells and transports important nutrients into them. Water cleanses and rids our body of toxins. It prevents kidney stone formation and constipation and keeps our body functioning at its best.

Scientific evidence shows that regular consumption of sugar sweetened beverages is associated with a higher risk of heart and vascular diseases in women, even after other unhealthful lifestyle or dietary factors were taken into consideration. [575]

Chapter 16 - The 12 Week Guerrilla Diet & Lifestyle Program

As I mentioned in Chapter 13, try bringing home a water dispenser. They come in all shapes and sizes to match any home and any budget. These water dispensers make drinking water so easy and convenient that it becomes difficult to ignore.

WEEK 3

This week choose a day and time and add two – 30 minute block of a chosen endurance exercise to your schedule.

In previous chapters I have shown the evidence suggesting that by increasing physical activity levels the health risks of obesity and other common modern world diseases are drastically reduced. In fact, physically active adults as well as children have a lower mortality risk than their unfit and inactive peers within the same body mass index groups. [576, 5767, 578] This importance of physical activity on our health is unwavering.

Today we have apps on our smart phones and watches that record the steps and the mileage we make a day without any effort on our part. All you have to do is have your smart phone handy with you and by the end of the day you will see how much you have walked. You may be surprised that you are actually walking more than you thought you were, however, in some cases, most of us are much less active than we should be. Previous hunter-gatherers were walking a minimum of 3.7 miles (six kilometers) per day and these are the minimum physical activity levels that we should be aiming for as well.

Use the stairs instead of the elevator, park your car further away from your destination to increase your daily walking/running distance, and take the long way instead of the short cut to reach your destination.

This week will you not only be more observant of your activity levels, you will add two – thirty minute uninterrupted exercise blocks to your weekly schedule. During these thirty minute exercise blocks, you can do any preferred endurance exercise like walking, biking, or swimming for a minimum of thirty minutes straight. Continuously and uninterruptedly walk around the mall during off-peak hours if unable to walk outside, find a local school track, go to your local park if the weather is fine, or you can choose to ride a bike to work. Any endurance exercise you do continuously for more than thirty minutes once a week is good. Try to fit it within your schedule to make it easier to adopt this practice. If you know that you will not have time to exercise after work, go walking with a coworker at lunch. If a continuous thirty minute walk seems boring to you, take your smartphone along with you so you can listen to interesting podcasts or music to make this time enjoyable for you.

It is important to keep in mind that anything new you start does not need to be love at first sight. The first endurance exercise program that you try does not need to be the best exercise option for you. Keep searching until you find the perfect match for you and your lifestyle, as long as you keep your once a week exercise block in check.

I use the "Health" app given for free with every iPhone 5 and subsequent models. Smart phone apps can also help you keep an activity journal to track your progress. This can be one of your most important tools for staying on a healthy path. By recording your progress you have a handy reminder of when you need to exercise which helps keep you focused, and also allows you to catch slip-ups in your schedule.

WEEK 4

This week, reduce added oils to your foods to a minimum.

Oils are processed foods, they go through an extraction phase removing the oil, typically from a seed, nut or fruit and then a refinement phase altering the appearance, texture, taste, smell, or stability of the oil to meet buyer expectations. Oil carries a high fat content with no other nutrient value. Oil has no minerals, vitamins, and no fiber. Oil contains high levels of inflammatory omega-6 fatty acids which increase inflammation and oxidative damage to the inner lining of all our blood vessels. [579, 580, 581] Synthetic oils which have a long shelf life also disrupt brain function and cellular function.

Chapter 16 - The 12 Week Guerrilla Diet & Lifestyle Program

This week remove fried foods from your menu. This includes removing French fries, removing deep-fried schnitzel, onion rings, fried fish including fish sticks, fried eggs, and all other fried meat products. Go for scrambled or preferably boiled eggs, oven baked organic chicken which has lower fat levels, baked vegetables, or home made stir fried vegetables using less than a tablespoon of coconut oil, and tomato based sauces instead of oil based sauces.

Once you reduce oils in your diet to a minimum and learn to cook fat free, you are immediately decreasing your risk of suffering from heart disease, stroke, and diabetes. You will also reduce your calorie intake immediately from fats and thereby increase the percentage of your diet which comes from more nutrient dense foods. In this way you will start to lose weight faster and reduce your risk from suffering the consequences of obesity.

Removing oils from the diet includes removing those from your salad dressing including olive oil. You can add flavor to your salads by adding a squeeze of lemon on top with a little garlic and mustard. You can also use sugar free balsamic vinegar as well as low salt soya sauce to add flavor if you desire. At first you may need time to get used to the taste, but slowly your taste buds will renew their affinity for natural flavors by carrying new messages from your tongue to the brain thereby creating new neural networks. This will slowly enable you to be more sensitive to the different tastes of foods and relearn to love the natural flavors that are less strong than their unnatural counterparts.

WEEK 5

From this moment on, choose whole grains instead of simple carbohydrates.

Make a real effort to eat only whole grain versions of breads, pasta, noodles, porridge, rice, any other carbohydrate rich dishes you consume.

Refined grains are unnaturally processed foods. They lead to rapid spikes in blood sugar levels which leads to insulin resistance and weight gain. Eating processed refined grains is known to increase the risk of many Western world diseases. [582, 583] The rapid absorption of glucose after consuming refined carbohydrates induces a sequence of hormonal and metabolic changes that promote excessive food intake in obese subjects. These foods actually increase appetite because the body is hungering for nutrients which it doesn't receive form these processed grains. (584)

When you consume whole grains you will also naturally increase your fiber intake. Fiber rich foods adjust the gut microbiome to induce weight loss and health as well as modifying leptin and other hormone production that regulate satiety and energy intake.

These bacteria also help us digest our foods (they ferment dietary fiber into short-chain fatty acids, such as acetic acid and butyric acid), which strengthens our gut wall, improving absorption of nutrients, and help us to lose weight by enhancing satiety). We have only 20 genes that encode for enzymes that digest carbohydrates, whereas one bacteria has 260 genes encoding for enzymes that break down carbohydrates.

Furthermore, lean individuals tend to have a wider variety of Bacteroidetes, a community of bacteria that break down bulky plant starches and fibers into shorter molecules that the body can use as a source of energy. Overweight individuals have less of these species. The more fiber consumed in the diet, the more the Bacteroidetes community will thrive, supporting our overall health and weight loss.

WEEK 6

This week reduce or preferably avoid chemically processed foods with refined ingredients and artificial substances.

The public and the food companies have known for decades now that processed foods are not good for us. However, food companies are still using scientific methods to get people hooked on chemically processed foods that are convenient and inexpensive. Processed foods with high levels of sugar or fructose corn syrup, fat, and salt which, when consumed in excess, are seriously harmful to our health are still being created on a daily basis. Modern research and even research dating back to the early 1980's support the role of sugar in the epidemics of metabolic syndrome, cancer, cardiovascular

Chapter 16 - The 12 Week Guerrilla Diet & Lifestyle Program

disease, and Type 2 diabetes, [584, 585, 586, 587, 588, 589, 590, 591, 592] and the role of fats and salt in raised blood pressure, heart disease, and stroke, [593] as well as diabetes since salt reduces insulin resistance. [594]

We are evolutionarily inclined to love these foods because they are necessary for survival. The food industry knows this and spends massive resources on making foods as palatable and as addictive as possible.

This week you will begin looking at food labels and remove from your diet high salt foods namely any that have over half a teaspoon (2.5 gm) of salt, as well as all foods products found in Chapter 13 under the two headings:
1. *"Consume Foods That Will Not Cause an Inflammatory Response."*
2. *"Consume Foods That Will Not Burden the Body."*

In the beginning you may feel that foods are too tasteless for you to enjoy because your taste buds have become used to the strong unnatural chemical flavors. In order to overcome this first period with as little cravings as possible, naturally increase salt rich vegetables to your meals. Salt-rich vegetables include celery, parsley, nori, seaweed, sage, kale, garlic, onion, and other sea vegetables.

You may also begin using a healthier version of the processed table salt which is the mineral rich Himalayan salt, or freshly mined salt which can be purchased at any health food store. These salts also contain small amounts of trace elements which in small amounts are generally good for human health.

WEEK 7

This week reduce the amount of animal products you eat by eating no more than 300 grams – 12 oz. of meat, eggs, and fish combined per week.

Choose two days during the week when you consume a low fat meat or fish dish of 150 g (6 oz.) at each meal. Stick to serving these items on the same days of the week as that will make it much

Chapter 16 - The 12 Week Guerrilla Diet & Lifestyle Program

simpler to follow through with on a long term basis. Adding an egg into this equation equals 50 g of animal fat and protein, and you should reduce your meat consumption by 50 g for every egg consumed in a week.

If you decide to go completely vegan for any reason, as I have, you will need to supplement your diet with methylcobalamine (an absorbable form of vitamin B12) on a bi-monthly basis or on a weekly basis depending on the type of supplement taken (liquid for or as a sublingual tablet). Pregnant women or women during their monthly menstruation should also supplement their diet with a natural, gentle iron supplement twice during their menstruation period and twice a week during pregnancy and lactation. Gentle iron supplements provide iron in the form of Iron Bis-Glycinate, a well-tolerated formula that prevents constipation.

To make this change easier, begin supplementing your diet with any form of nuts or seeds. You can snack on natural, unsalted, and unroasted nuts, or you may add seeds sprinkled to your food or in the form of a spread to your sandwiches. Tasty sandwich and cracker spreads include sesame seed spread (tahini), natural unroasted peanut butter, cashew, or almond spreads.

In Chapter 6 of this book I went into great detail and covered much research of how eating high levels of animal products is directly linked to the development of many modern day diseases including cancer, diabetes, rheumatoid arthritis, heart and vascular diseases, and a number of other illnesses. Reduction of dietary animal products has shown to stop or even reverse the progression of some cancers. [5945, 5956, 597] Furthermore, people consuming high levels of animal meat have been shown to die prematurely more frequently than those consuming lower levels. [598]

Research also shows that consuming a mostly plant-based diet minimizes or even eliminates a person's genetic inclination for developing chronic diseases, such as Type 2 diabetes, cardiovascular disease, and cancer. [599, 600, 601, 602, 603, 604, 605] Animal products switch on genes which increase visceral fat storage (in your belly) which raises the risk for modern Western world chronic diseases. [606]

Saturated fat also activates genes that increase inflammation while turning off cancer-fighting genes at the same time. (607)

WEEK 8

This week add one more 30 minute endurance exercise block or walking routine to your weekly schedule, followed by a 15 minute muscle building strength program to help sculpt your body.

After completing your third weekly endurance exercise, I would like you to add the following strength program to help sculpt your body.

Perform the next five simple strength exercises either in a gym or at home using home barbells or anything that can easily be grasped that weigh 1–6 kg (2–13 pounds) according to your current physical ability. These are whole body workouts working on all major muscle groups.

Perform three sets of ten repetitions each for each of the five strength exercises below. Focus on raising and lowering your weights and holding your body in a controlled manner.

To see the exercises below performed, please visit the link below:

https://goo.gl/0Ittzb

1. **Squat to Overhead Press**. This exercise works leg quadriceps and hamstring muscles, bottom gluteus maximus muscles, abdominal muscles, and shoulder muscles.
    1. Hold a hand weight of 1–6 kg (2–13 pound weight) in each hand held at chest height, palms facing forward.
    2. Stand with feet shoulder-width apart with elbows bent.
    3. Lower into a squat position, making sure your knees do not bend forward over your toe line. Hold for a moment.
    4. Straighten your knees to stand up while raising the weights above you head.
    5. Return to starting position and repeat.

2. **Step with Bicep Curl**. This exercise works leg quadriceps and hamstring muscles, bottom gluteus maximus muscles, abdominal muscles, and hand biceps muscles.
   1. Stand with one foot on a sturdy bench or low step, holding a weight in each hand.
   2. Lift yourself up to standing on the step. At the same time, curl weights up toward shoulders.
   3. Go back down and raise your other leg on the step.
   4. Again, lift yourself up to standing on the step. At the same time, curl weights up toward shoulders.
   5. Switch sides and repeat.
3. **Triceps Press**. This exercise works on all three of the triceps muscles, shoulder, abdomen and back stabilizing muscles.
   1. Get into a plank position with your toes resting on a stair, table, or ball. Place your hands a little closer than shoulder-width apart.
   2. Bend your arms slowly until your elbows reach a 90-degree angle.
   3. Press back up to straighten.
   4. Return to starting position and repeat.
4. **Superman**. This exercise works the back and bottom gluteus maximus muscles.
   1. Lie face down with arms and legs extended, toes pointed, palms down.
   2. Inhale while raising arms and legs as high as you can; pause.
   3. Exhale while slowly returning to starting position.
5. **Abdominal Curls.** This exercise works on your abdominal muscles.
   1. Lie down with your knees bent and your feet placed flat on the ground.
   2. Place your hands either behind your head or on opposing shoulders by crossing your hands over your chest.
   3. Tighten your abdominal muscles and then slowly lift your head and then your shoulder blades off the floor until you reach a 75-degree angle.

4. Slowly bring your back to the floor in a slightly arched fashion.
5. Repeat.

WEEK 9

This week you will begin reprogramming of your mind to help you form and keep new and beneficial habits more easily.

This week we will focus on mind work and not change anything about your diet, but instead help change your mindset.

Your job this week is to watch a subliminal mind film I have created especially for you, twice daily. (You can find these mind films inside the Guerrilla Diet Online Training Program).

Lie down in a comfortable spot and watch the film. After viewing the film, I would like you to envision yourself reaching your very pleasurable end goal that you desire to be and that you created for yourself in Chapter 10 under the heading *"Raising Your Chances of Succeeding at Dieting."* This film allows you to align your thoughts with your new reality and then your action will soon to follow, aligning themselves up with your new reality as well.

This week you also have the chance to make yourself post-it notes to hang on your computer, your bathroom mirror, and in your car with a mission statement that is in present tense of what you wish to achieve. For example, "I weigh 60 kg". "I am happy, energetic and beautiful!", "I am radiating with health and energy!", "I lose weight easily while eating tasty foods."

I also recommend adding a desired action to your mission statement that you will be able to do once you have reached your goal. For example, "I'm wearing a bathing suit on my holiday and many people are gazing at me because I look so great." Or "I am wearing my beautiful 'X' and fit into it perfectly!"

Also this week during your chosen endurance exercise, I would like you to focus your thoughts, visualize and repeat your mission statement end goal and your desired action twice weekly and in present tense, as if you already own it.

Chapter 16 - The 12 Week Guerrilla Diet & Lifestyle Program

This week's mind exercise may not seem very important at first, and may feel to some like a wasted week, but this is not the case. It is important at this stage to help your brain form new neural networks as new skills and habits are formed. This week is very important for your success towards the achievement of your goal!

WEEK 10

This week remove dairy products from your diet and try out sprouting and increasing lentil and bean consumption instead.

This week I would like you to make all the effort to reduce most, or all, of the dairy products you consume in your diet.

In Chapter 7, I covered the health and weight loss problems that come along with consuming milk products beyond the age of infancy in 75% of the world's population, as well as the nutrient deficits they lead to in all populations. Dairy products are proven to increase feelings of anxiety due to their effects on other nutrient stores as well as increasing risk for heart disease, cancer, cataracts, osteoporosis, and diabetes.

Good, non-dairy sources of calcium can be found in the chart in Chapter 13 under the heading *"Consume Foods Rich in Both Calcium and Magnesium."*

There are many dishes that have milk substitutes and they are quite easy to come by. You can exchange dairy milk for soy, coconut, almond, oat, or even rice milk. They all taste good and can take the place of milk in your breakfast muesli or in your tea or coffee.

To help you in your effort to reduce or remove dairy products, add more lentils or beans to your diet.

Lentils are an excellent source of minerals. They are also rich in dietary soluble fiber which helps stabilize blood sugar levels, especially important if you suffer from insulin resistance, hypoglycemia, or diabetes. Lentils are also rich in insoluble fiber which helps balance blood sugar levels by providing a slow and steady energy source. [608] Lentils are also rich in copper, phosphorus, and manganese, and have high levels of iron, protein, vitamin B1, pantothenic acid, zinc, potassium, and vitamin B6. Lentils are rich in complex carbohydrates, sodium, fatty acids, and protein, [609, 610] and are therefore a very highly recommended food source. Beans are similar to lentils, but are slightly higher in fiber and slightly lower in minerals yet are also a highly recommended food source. There are so many types of lentils and beans to add variety to your diet and diversity to your nutrient consumption.

By consuming lentils and beans you will no doubt quickly remove any cravings to consume dairy products, help yourself easily and quickly lose weight, and feel good more than you imagine. Sprouting, which increases the availability of minerals, vitamins, and enzymes in the food will also help remove dairy product cravings.

WEEK 11

This week reduce plain sugar consumption to an absolute minimum.

To help you with any sweet tooth you may still be having, choose any type of fruit or dried fruit instead of sugar rich foods. They are real convenience foods without the negative effects of processed convenience foods and are easy to eat and carry around.

You may also include chocolate made with a minimum of 85% cocoa if you have a real urge for chocolate. Sugar substitutes including Maltitol and Xylitol are sugar alcohols, which have 75-90% of the sweetness of sugar but half of its calories. These are not highly recommended alternatives although they do not promote tooth decay as sugar does and have a somewhat lesser effect on blood sugar levels. They are not recommended because they harm the beneficial gut microbes that maintain health and support weight loss.

The stevia plant is the best sugar substitute. Stevia comes from an herb found in Central and South America that is up to 40 times sweeter than sugar, but has zero calories and doesn't affect blood sugar levels. Stevia has a bitter aftertaste, but you may solve this problem by growing the plant on your windowsill and choose the sweetest parts to sweeten food.

Chapter 16 - The 12 Week Guerrilla Diet & Lifestyle Program

The fact is that removing sugar will come much more easily after you have changed your diet to consume more whole grain complex carbohydrates and protein rich lentils and beans, all of which help stabilize blood sugar levels. High consumption of refined sugar causes insulin resistance and predisposes a person for a fatty liver. Scientific evidence shows strong links between sugar consumption and obesity, diabetes, heart disease and stroke. [613, 614, 615, 616] Sugar also stimulates the expression of genes that produce fat, keeping us overweight bombarding our weight loss efforts. [617]

As a side note: I recommend you eat whole fruits separately from all other carbohydrate-rich foods (have at least 1-2 hours after a meal before you consume fruits) so that you won't be consuming too much fructose together with glucose which leads to deposition of fat in the liver leading to inflammation and chronic diseases. In other words, I recommend that you stop consuming fruits as a dessert and eat them only between meals. Choose nuts, seeds or dark chocolate as healthy dessert alternatives.

WEEK 12

This week go on regular intermittent fasts at least five days a week.

After understanding the benefits of intermittent fasting in Chapter 13 guideline number 16, I would like you to make the last change in lifestyle change and this involves fasting intermittently at least five days a week.

The fast I recommend lasts for 12-13 hours, from the last meal consumed at night to the first meal eaten in the day. No matter when you finished your last meal, eat your first meal (breakfast) no earlier than twelve hours later and no later than thirteen hours later.

Now I know that for some it may seem difficult to stop eating for prolonged hours. It was difficult for me at first. This is why it's important for me to mention that hunger is an adaptive response, meaning that the body adapts to an environmental demand. Once your body gets used to this pattern of eating and then fasting, this new habit will become easy to commit to and will provide you with many health benefits.

Chapter 17

A 30 Day Example of The Guerrilla Diet and Lifestyle Program

"Strength is the capacity to break a chocolate bar into four pieces with your bare hands – and then eat just one of the pieces."

– Judith Viorst

In this chapter you will get some small additional tips and a 30 day example for implementing **The Guerrilla Diet and Lifestyle Program** to help you achieve your health and weight loss goals easily.

Regarding Breakfast

First thing in the morning squeeze one whole, (or half), of a lemon into a cup and drink it in one shot. This ritual reduces hunger almost completely and as a bonus will make you completely forget what a sore throat ever felt like. Following the lemon juice ritual, drink as many glasses of water as you need in order to feel rehydrated (normally 1-3 glasses depending on the room temperature in the night).

Chapter 17 - A 30 Day Example of The Guerrilla Diet and Lifestyle Program

Breakfast is a very important meal and through my personal experience and my extensive studies in the field of nutrition, I recommend eating breakfast only when you start to feel hungry in the morning and not earlier. Eat breakfast twelve hours after you have finished eating dinner. Breakfast should be easy and quick to prepare. Once you start feeling hungry, and after twelve hours of fasting, breakfast should be available for you within minutes so that you do not find yourself grabbing any unhealthy alternative just because you are too hungry to wait until something fits prepared. The moment you start to feel hungry, eat the breakfast that you prepared earlier. The idea is to prevent the breakdown of protein tissue for supplying your body with its energy needs, therefore it is important to begin the day with a carbohydrate rich meal with plenty of fiber.

Regarding Lunch and Dinner

Regarding lunch and dinner, try to fill your plate so that 35% of each meal is composed of vegetables, preferably with some green leafy type as well as vegetables that are rich in prebiotics to maintain a healthy gut bacteria composition that will help reduce fat absorption. You may choose to cover the base of your plate with leafy greens to allow them to gain some flavor from your other foods and a dash of any type of onion or garlic as a spice.

Eat the meals when you are hungry, no matter the time of day. If you feel you need to eat your lunch at 11:30 am, then by all means do so. If you are not hungry at 7:00 pm, then wait to eat your dinner until you do feel hungry, but have it prepared and ready to eat so that when feelings of hunger appear you will have something within easy access to feed on.

Snacks should be eaten between meals. However, if you are feeling very hungry, opt to eat the meal itself, even if a little sooner than usual, to avoid consuming too much food during snack time.

Chapter 17 - A 30 Day Example of The Guerrilla Diet and Lifestyle Program

Regarding Your Exercise Routine

During weeks 1 and 2, maintain the level of exercise you had a before committing to **The Guerrilla Diet and Lifestyle Program.**

During weeks 3 and 5, add two – 30 minute exercise block a week to your regular physical activity levels.

During weeks 5 and 8, add three – 30 minute exercise blocks a week to your regular physical activity levels with one strength training exercise block.

During weeks 8 and 12, add three – 30 minute exercise blocks a week to your regular physical activity levels with two strength training exercise blocks.

Immediately after exercising, try to eat a meal. Remember that ancient humans were physically active before they found a place to stop and forage. This habit helps replenish muscle glycogen stores and heal muscle tissue more quickly.

Mind reprogramming should also be done regularly a minimum of twice daily, even for a short period, to keep you focused on your goals and to help you reach them as soon as possible.

A 30 Day Example of The Guerrilla Diet and Lifestyle Program

In the chart on the following pages you have a 30 day example of *The Guerrilla Diet and Lifestyle Program*.

You can find free Guerrilla Diet recipes on my blog below:

TheGuerrillaDiet.com/blog

Or order my book: ***Best Way To Lose Weight - A Step By Step Guide To Lose Weight In a Month The Guerrilla Diet Way***
Complete with precise health promoting recipes, snacks, weight loss supplements and exercise programs as well as two very valuable special bonuses.

Chapter 17 - A 30 Day Example of The Guerrilla Diet and Lifestyle Program

Check it out here:

TheGuerrillaDiet.com/the-guerrilla-diet/lose-weight-in-a-month/

or on Amazon here: **http://amzn.to/1L72vvp**

☑ = Easy and quick recipes

Table 12: A 30 Day Example of The Guerrilla Diet and Lifestyle Program

	Breakfast	**Lunch**	**Dinner**	**☑ Snacks between meals**	**Exercise days**
Day 1	☑ 1 whole wheat pita with almond butter and sugar free natural fruit jam	1-2 cups of brown rice served with orange lentil and vegetable soup	☑ Pasta from corn or durum wheat with tomato pea and spinach sauce	Summer – apricot Winter – apple + a handful of macadamia nuts	
Day 2	☑ 2 cups of sugar free natural Muesli with almond milk	Brown and wild rice and small black lentils seved with salad	☑ Whole wheat bread with a plate of natural hummus and oil free fried Shiitake mushroom	Summer – 1 cup of berries Winter – clementine + a handful of hazelnuts	Exercise day (weeks 2- onward)

Chapter 17 - A 30 Day Example of The Guerrilla Diet and Lifestyle Program

Table 12: A 30 Day Example of The Guerrilla Diet and Lifestyle Program

	Breakfast	Lunch	Dinner	☑ Snacks between meals	Exercise days
Day 3	☑ Whole wheat bagel with sesame paste		Vegan sushi	Summer – plum Winter – orange + a handful of Almonds	
Day 4	☑ Whole oats with flax, chia, pumpkin and ☑ sunflower seeds with oat milk	Brown round rice risotto and asparagus	☑ Arabic salad with whole wheat bread, olives and tahini or sesame paste	Summer – 1 cup of strawberries Winter – pear + a handful of Brazil nuts	Exercise day (weeks 2- onward)
Day 5	☑ Whole wheat toast with avocado sprinkled with sunflower seeds	Brown basmati rice with white beans and bamia	200 g fat free steak, or egg served with salad and new potatoes	Summer – 2 figs Winter – 2 dates + a handful of Pistachios	

Chapter 17 - A 30 Day Example of The Guerrilla Diet and Lifestyle Program

Table 12: A 30 Day Example of The Guerrilla Diet and Lifestyle Program

	Breakfast	Lunch	Dinner	☑ Snacks between meals	Exercise days
Day 6	Healthy pancakes	Magadra – with tahini salad	☑ Vegan lentil burger with whole wheat bun	Summer – grapefruit Winter – nectarine + a handful of Cashews	Exercise day (weeks 8- onward)
Day 7	☑ fruit salad sprinkled with chia and flax seeds	Baked Potato topped with corn served with salad	Whole-wheat spaghetti and aubergine and tomato sauce with peas	banana + a handful of unfrosted peanuts	
Day 8	☑ Bran-flakes with dairy free milk	Vegan chili con carne served on brown rice	☑ Sweet potatoes and beetroot salad	Summer – peach Winter – apple + a handful of walnuts	

Chapter 17 - A 30 Day Example of The Guerrilla Diet and Lifestyle Program

Table 12: A 30 Day Example of The Guerrilla Diet and Lifestyle Program

	Breakfast	Lunch	Dinner	☑ Snacks between meals	Exercise days
Day 9	☑ 2 small bananas and 7 cashew nuts	Butter beans and cauliflower served on millet	Whole wheat pearl barley with artichoke bottoms and green beans	Summer – 1 cup of watermelon Winter – clementine + a handful of Cashews	Exercise day (weeks 2- onward)
Day 10	☑ 1 Whole-wheat matzo with peanut butter and sugar free natural fruit jam	rice noodles with shelled edamame and bean sprouts	☑ Mashed potatoes and yellow beans with spinach	1 cup of pomegranate seeds + a handful of Brazil nuts	
Day 11	☑ 4 Rice crackers and avocado with sesame paste	Tricolored rice and red lentil soup	Whole-wheat couscous with chickpea and vegetable soup	Summer – cherry Winter – pear + a handful of Pecans	Exercise day (weeks 2- onward)

Chapter 17 - A 30 Day Example of The Guerrilla Diet and Lifestyle Program

Table 12: A 30 Day Example of The Guerrilla Diet and Lifestyle Program

	Breakfast	**Lunch**	**Dinner**	☑ **Snacks between meals**	**Exercise days**
Day 12	Tofu scramble	Millet and black eyed peas stew served with chopped vegetable salad	☑ Buckwheat noodles with snow peas and asparagus	Summer – apricot Winter – apple + 2 cups of coconut water	
Day 13	☑ Whole spelt bread with hazelnut butter and apple sauce	Brown lentils in coconut milk, served on brown basmati rice	200 g steamed fish, with kale and new potatoes	Summer – 1 cup of berries Winter – pear + a handful of unfrosted peanuts	Exercise day (weeks 8- onward)
Day 14	☑ 2 cups of sugar-free natural Muesli with almond milk	Yellow lentils with chard, served on red Indian rice	☑ Aubergine salad, and whole wheat bread	1 cup of pomegranate seeds + a handful of Pistachios	

Chapter 17 - A 30 Day Example of The Guerrilla Diet and Lifestyle Program

Table 12: A 30 Day Example of The Guerrilla Diet and Lifestyle Program

	Breakfast	Lunch	Dinner	☑ Snacks between meals	Exercise days
Day 15	☑ Whole wheat bagel with sesame paste and sugar free natural fruit jam	Whole tri-color Quinoa Tabouli	☑ Buckwheat noodles with stir fried vegetables	Summer – 1 cup of raspberries Winter – clementine + a handful of hazelnuts	
Day 16	☑ fruit salad sprinkled with chia and flax seeds	Millet and chickpea tahini	☑ Whole wheat bread with a plate of natural hummus and oil free fried Shiitake mushrooms	Summer – plum Winter – orange + a handful of Almonds	Exercise day (weeks 2- onward)
Day 17	☑ Bran flakes with non dairy milk	Whole wheat pasta with Mushrooms and black beans	Vegan sushi	Summer – peach Winter – apple + a handful of Walnuts	

Chapter 17 - A 30 Day Example of The Guerrilla Diet and Lifestyle Program

Table 12: A 30 Day Example of The Guerrilla Diet and Lifestyle Program

	Breakfast	**Lunch**	**Dinner**	☑ **Snacks between meals**	**Exercise days**
Day 18	☑ Corn tortilla with avocado sprinkled with sunflower seeds	Vegan meatballs and whole-wheat spaghetti	☑ Pasta from corn or durum wheat with tomato pea and spinach sauce	Summer – 1 cup of watermelon Winter – clementine + a handful of Macadamia nuts	Exercise day (weeks 2- onward)
Day 19	☑ Whole oats with flax, chia, pumpkin and sunflower seeds with rice milk	Stir fry tofu and veg served with brown round rice	200 g steamed fish, with kale and new potatoes	Summer – 1 cup of berries Winter – pear + a handful of Brazil Nuts	
Day 20	☑ Whole-wheat bagel with sesame paste	Yellow lentils with chard, served on wild rice	Whole wheat penne pasta with tomato and pea sauce	Banana + a handful of Pecans	Exercise day (weeks 8- onward)

Chapter 17 - A 30 Day Example of The Guerrilla Diet and Lifestyle Program

Table 12: A 30 Day Example of The Guerrilla Diet and Lifestyle Program

	Breakfast	Lunch	Dinner	☑ Snacks between meals	Exercise days
Day 21	☑ 4 Buckwheat crackers and avocado with sesame paste	Quinoa and cannellini bean burger, served with salad	☑ Vegan rice and chia burger with whole-wheat bun	Summer – plum Winter – orange + a handful of Cashews	
Day 22	☑ 2 small bananas and 7 cashew nuts	Bean stew served with whole grain pearl barley	☑ Arabic salad with whole wheat bread, olives and tahini or sesame paste	1 cup of pomegranate seeds + a handful of unfrosted peanuts	
Day 23	Healthy pancakes	Brown lentils in coconut milk, served on Brown basmati rice	Whole wheat spaghetti and aubergine and tomato sauce with peas	Summer – apricot Winter – apple + 2 cups coconut water	Exercise day (weeks 2- onward)

Chapter 17 - A 30 Day Example of The Guerrilla Diet and Lifestyle Program

Table 12: A 30 Day Example of The Guerrilla Diet and Lifestyle Program

	Breakfast	Lunch	Dinner	☑ Snacks between meals	Exercise days
Day 24	☑ 1 Whole wheat matzo with hazelnut butter and 100% fruit jam	Whole wheat noodles with broccoli and pine nuts	☑ Sweet potatoes with fennel in the oven and beetroot salad	Summer – grape-fruit Winter – nectarine + a handful of Pistachios	
Day 25	Tofu scramble	Magadra served with salad	Whole-wheat barley with artichoke bottoms and green beans	Summer – 1 cup of strawberries Winter – pear + a handful of hazelnuts	Exercise day (weeks 2- onward)
Day 26	☑ 1 whole wheat Pita with almond butter and sugar free natural fruit jam	Stir fry tofu and veg served with brown round rice	☑ Mashed potatoes and asparagus with corn	Dried pineapple + a handful of Almonds	

Chapter 17 - A 30 Day Example of The Guerrilla Diet and Lifestyle Program

Table 12: A 30 Day Example of The Guerrilla Diet and Lifestyle Program

	Breakfast	Lunch	Dinner	☑ Snacks between meals	Exercise days
Day 27	☑ 4 Rice crackers and avocado with sesame paste	Whole tri-color Quinoa Tabouli	Whole-wheat couscous with chickpea and veg soup	Summer – 2 figs Winter – 2 dates + a handful of walnuts	Exercise day (weeks 8- onward)
Day 28	☑ Corn tortilla with avocado sprinkled with sunflower seeds	Whole-wheat noodles with broccoli and pine nuts	200 g steamed fish, with spinach and new potatoes	Summer – 1 cup of cherries Winter – apple + a handful of Macademia nuts	
Day 29	☑ Whole oats with flax, chia, hazelnuts and dates served with coconut milk	Quinoa and cannellini bean burger, served with salad	☑ Whole wheat spaghetti and ☑ artichoke with tomato sauce and pine kernels	Summer – 1 cup of water-melon Winter – clementine + a handful of Brazil nuts	

Chapter 17 - A 30 Day Example of The Guerrilla Diet and Lifestyle Program

	Breakfast	Lunch	Dinner	☑ Snacks between meals	Exercise days
Day 30				+ 2 cups coconut water	Exercise day (weeks 2- onward)

Table 12: A 30 Day Example of The Guerrilla Diet and Lifestyle Program

A Personal Message:

Please remember: even if you have not lost all of the weight you desired to lose during the twelve weeks, you will continue to lose all of the weight you desire even if you only follow 80% of the recommendations in this book. I promise you that if you just keep at it you will reach your desired weight in due time.
Wishing you the best of luck in becoming happy and healthy.

Galit Goldfarb

If you would like in depth coaching with this diet, please feel free to join my online training program "***The Guerrilla Diet Bootcamp***".

Since you've purchased this book, I'm offering you a 50% discount for enrolling in the Guerrilla Diet & Lifestyle Online Training Program. This course will help you easily put together the pieces and get you on the way to a new slim, trim and healthier you. The link below will take you to a page to insert your personal details and you will receive a 50% off coupon to redeem when registering for the course.

https://goo.gl/v87JYI

For those of you who have enjoyed the book but prefer an individual touch with small group mentoring calls to get you quickly into the process of losing weight and achieving the health that you deserve for good with added personal touch, I have a group coached programs with only a few participants designed especially for you. These coached programs are offered a few times a year. Please visit ***The Guerrilla Diet and Lifestyle Program*** website (www.TheGuerillaDiet.com) to find out when the next coached online program begins.

For those who prefer one-on-one private coaching sessions, please visit: **TheGuerrillaDiet.com/consult-2**
For any questions or support, just mail us at:
support@theguerrilladiet.com or write to us on Facebook:
https://www.facebook.com/theguerrilladiet/

Chapter 18

References

Without the hard work of the following people, this book would never have been possible.

1. Cynthia L. Ogden, Margaret D. Carroll, Brian K. Kit, Katherine M. Flegal. JAMA. 2014;311(8):806-814. doi:10.1001/jama.2014.732.
2. CDC National Center for Health Statistics. Adult Obesity Facts.
3. NHLBI Global Health Strategic Plan 2012-2017, Office of Global Health; National Heart, Lung, and Blood Institute
4. Sharon Begley. As America's waistline expands, costs soar. Reuters New York; Apr 30, (2012)
5. Jeffrey Levi, Laura M. Segal, MA, Rebecca St. Laurent, JD ,Albert Lang, Jack Rayburn. F as in Fat: How obesity threatens Americas future. Trust for America's Health. The Robert Wood Johnson Foundation Report. (2012)
6. Boston Medical Center Nutrition Services and Weight Management
7. Aylwyn Scally et al; Insights into hominid evolution from the gorilla genome sequence; Nature; 2012; 483, 169–175 doi:10.1038/nature10842
8. Aylwyn Scally, Julien Y. Dutheil, LaDeana W. Hillier, Gregory E. Jordan, Ian Goodhead, Javier Herrero, Asger Hobolth, Tuuli Lappalainen, Thomas Mailund, Tomas
9. Marques-Bonet, Shane McCarthy, Stephen H. Montgomery, Petra C. Schwalie, Y. Amy Tang, Michelle C. Ward, Yali Xue,
10. Bryndis Yngvadottir, Can Alkan, Lars N. Andersen, Qasim Ayub, Edward V. Ball, Kathryn Beal, Brenda J. Bradley, Yuan Chen, Chris M. Clee et al. Insights into hominid evolution from the gorilla genome sequence. Nature. 2012; 483, 169–175 doi:10.1038/nature10842
11. Goidts V, Armengol L, Schempp W et al. Identification of large-scale human-specific copy number differences by inter-species array

References

12. comparative genomic hybridization. Hum. Genet. 2006;119 (1–2): 185–98. doi:10.1007/s00439-005-0130-9. PMID 16395594.
13. Zeng, J, et al. 2012. Divergent Whole-Genome Methylation Maps of Human and Chimpanzee Brains Reveal Epigenetic Basis of Human Regulatory Evolution. American Journal of Human Genetics. 91 (3): 455-465.
14. Glazko GV, Nei M. Estimation of divergence times for major lineages of primate species. Mol. Biol. Evol. 2003;20 (3): 424–34. doi:10.1093/molbev/msg050. PMID 12644563
15. Cynthia L. Ogden, Cheryl D. Fryar. Margaret D. Carroll, Katherine M. Flegal. Mean Body Weight, Height, and Body Mass Index, United States 1960–2002; Division of Health and Nutrition Examination Surveys
16. Donahue S M. Trends in birth weight and gestational length among singleton term births in the United States: 1990-2005. Obstetrics & Gynecology. 2010; 115: 2: 1: 357-64.
17. Cawthorn Lang KA. Primate factsheets: Gorilla (Gorilla) taxonomy, morphology & ecology. (2005)
18. Total energy expenditure (TEE) and physical activity levels (PAL) in adults: doubly-labelled water data". Energy and Protein requirements, Proceedings of an IDECG workshop. United Nations University. 1994-11-04. Retrieved 2014-11-10.
19. Herculano-Houzel S, Kaas JH. Not all brains are made the same: new views on brain scaling in evolution. Brain Behav Evol; 2011; 77(1): 33-44.
20. Herculano-Houzel. The human brain in numbers: a linearly scaled-up primate brain. Hum Neurosci. 2009; 3:31.
21. ZME Science; MIND & BRAIN, NEUROLOGY, STUDIES; Cooking food helped early humans grow bigger brains
22. Schmidt-Nielsen K. Scaling: Why Is Animal Size so important? Cambridge: Cambridge University Press; 1984.
23. Martin RP. Primate origins and evolution: a phylogenetic reconstruction. Princeton: Princeton University Press; 1990.
24. Bonner JT. Why size matters: from bacteria to blue whales. Princeton: Princeton University Press; 2006
25. Gorilla Walks Like A Man at British Animal Park (Video) Gather News Channel by Doug York on January 27, 2011
26. Encyclopædia Britannica, Gorilla, 7-3-2014
27. SeaWorld Parks & Entertainment; Gorillas Diet & Eating Habits
28. Haenel H. Phylogenesis and nutrition. Nahrung 1989; 33 (9): 867–87. PMID 2697806.

References

29. Cordain, Loren. Implications of Plio-pleistocene diets for modern humans. In Peter S. Ungar. Evolution of the human diet: the known, the unknown and the unknowable. pp. 264–5. (2007)
30. Earliest agriculture in the Americas Earliest cultivation of barley Earliest cultivation of figs – URLs retrieved November 19, 2014
31. Ulijaszek SJ. Human eating behaviour in an evolutionary ecological context. Proc Nutr Soc; November 2002; 61 (4): 517–26. doi:10.1079/PNS2002180. PMID 12691181.
32. Holden C, Mace R. Phylogenetic analysis of the evolution of lactose digestion in adults. Hum. Biol. October 1997;69 (5): 605–28. PMID 9299882.
33. Peyer, B. Comparative Odontology. Chicago: University of Chicago Press, 1968.
34. Humans Have Canine Teeth but Their Use Matters The Most: www.tonehealth.org/Do-Humans-Have-Canine-Teeth.htm
35. Charles Darwin. The descent of man (1871)
36. Maina, J. N. Functional Morphology of the Vertebrate Respiratory Systems. Enfield, New Hampshire: Science Publishers, (2002), p. 60.
37. Eva Bianconi, Allison Piovesan, Federica Facchin, Alina Beraudi, Raffaella Casadei, Flavia Frabetti, Lorenza Vitale, Maria Chiara Pelleri, Simone Tassani, Francesco Piva, Soledad Perez-Amodio, Pierluigi Strippoli, and Silvia Canaider. An estimation of the number of cells in the human body; Annals of Human Biology; 2013; Vol. 40, No. 6 , Pages 463-471 (doi:10.3109/03014460.2013.807878)
38. Von Koenigswald, G. H. R. Meeting Prehistoric Man. Lowe & Brydone (printers) LTD, London, Scientific Book Club Edition, 1956.
39. Popovich, D. G., Jenkins, D. J. A., Kendall, C. W. C., Dierenfeld, E. S., Carroll, R. W., Tariq, N., et al. The Western Lowland Gorilla Diet Has Implications for the Health of Humans and Other Hominoids. J. Nutr; 1997; 127,10, 2000-2005.
40. Stevens, C. E. & Hume. Comparative Physiology of the Vertebrate Digestive System, 2nd ed. p. 75. Cambridge University Press, Cambridge, UK. (1995)
41. Stevens and Hume, Comparative Physiology of the Vertebrate Digestive System. Cambridge; Cambridge University Press (1995)
42. Darwin, Charles. The Descent of Man, and selection in relation to sex. John Murray: (1871) London.
43. "Fascinating Baby Brains." Live Science. Accessed: November 14, 2014.
44. NI McNeil. The contribution of the large intestine to energy supplies in man. Am J Clin Nutr;1984; vol. 39 no. 2 338-342

References

45. Encyclopædia Britannica, Gorilla, 7-3-2014
46. Smith, Roff. "Oldest Known Hearth Found in Israel Cave". National Geographic. (2014)
47. National geographic Lowland Gorilla: animals.nationalgeographic.com/animals/mammals/lowland-gorilla/?source=A-to-Z
48. Kecmanovic, D. The paranoid attitude as the common form of social behavior. Sociologija, 1969; 11(4), 573-585.7
49. WHO Life expectancy". WHO. apps.who.int/gho/data/node.main.688?lang=en
50. Oded Galor and Omer Moav. Natural Selection and the Evolution of Life Expectancy. (2005)
51. Caspari, Rachel & Lee, Sang-Hee. Older age becomes common late in human evolution. Proceedings of the National Academy of Sciences; 2004; 101 (20): 10895–10900. doi:10.1073/pnas.0402857101. PMC 503716. PMID 15252198.
52. Steve Jones, Robert Martin & David Pilbeam. The Cambridge Encyclopedia of Human Evolution. Cambridge: Cambridge University Press. (1994) p. 242. ISBN 0-521-32370-3. Also ISBN 0-521-46786-1
53. CIA—The World Factbook—Rank Order—Life expectancy at birth
54. CDC. "Ten great public health achievements—United States, 1900–1999". JAMA; 1999; 281 ,16, 1481.
55. Zoo Gorillas Go Heart-Healthy with New Diet
56. McGuire J. T., Dierenfeld E. S., Poppenga R. H., Braselton W. E. Plasma alpha-tocopherol, retinol, cholesterol, and mineral concentrations in captive gorillas. J. Med. Primatol; 1989; 18:155–161.
57. Cousins, D. Mortality factors in captive gorillas. International Zoo News; 1979; 30:5-17.
58. Williamson E. Behavioural ecology of western lowland gorillas in Gabon. University of Stirling, Stirling (1988)
59. National Zoological Park, Smithsonian Institution fact-gorilla: nationalzoo.si.edu/animals/primates/facts/fact-gorilla.cfm
60. Haslam DW, James WP. "Obesity". Lancet; October 2005; 366 (9492): 1197–209. doi:10.1016/S0140-6736(05)67483-1. PMID 16198769.
61. U.S. Department of Health and Human Services. Overweight and obesity: a major public health issue. Prevention Report; 2001;16.
62. WVDHHR - Obesity, facts, figures and guidelines
63. Clinical guidelines on the identification, evaluation, and treatment of overweight and obesity in adults. Executive summary. National

References

Institutes of Health, National Heart, Lung, and Blood Institute, (June 1998).
64. Centre for disease Control, 50th Anniversary Report on Smoking and Health: www.cdc.gov/features/2014smokingreport/index.html
65. ACSPC - 2014 Cancer Facts & Figures report: www.cancer.org/acs/groups/content/@research/documents/webcontent/acspc-042151.pdf
66. Murphy SL, Xu JQ, Kochanek KD. Deaths: Final data for 2010. Natl Vital Stat Rep; 2013;61,4.
67. Jonah, Brian. A. Accident Risk and Risk-Taking Behavior among Young Drivers. Accident Analysis & Prevention;1986; 18:255–271.
68. Kraemer, Sebastian. The Fragile Male. British Medical Journal; 2000; 321:1609–1612.
69. Sahney, Sarda. "Recovery from the most profound mass extinction of all time" (PDF). Proceedings of the Royal Society B (London: Royal Society); 2008; 275 (1636): 759–765. doi:10.1098/rspb.2007.1370. ISSN 0962-8452. PMC 2596898. PMID 18198148
70. Chiappe, Luis M.; . "The Mesozoic Radiation of Birds". Annual Review of Ecology and Systematics (Palo Alto, CA: Annual Reviews); 2002; 33: 91–124. doi:10.1146/annurev.ecolsys.33.010802.150517. ISSN 1545-2069.
71. Rey LV, Holtz, Jr TR. Dinosaurs: the most complete, up-to-date encyclopaedia for dinosaur lovers of all ages. New York: Random House. (2007) ISBN 0-375-82419-7.
72. Dawkins, R. The Ancestor's Tale: A Pilgrimage to the Dawn of Evolution, Houghton Mifflin Harcourt, (2005) ISBN 978-0-618-61916-0
73. Wikipedia - Timeline of human evolution: en.m.wikipedia.org/wiki/Timeline_of_human_evolution
74. Groves, C. P.Wilson, D. E.; Reeder, D. M, eds. Mammal Species of the World (3rd ed.). Baltimore: Johns Hopkins University Press. (2005) pp. 181–184. OCLC 62265494. ISBN 0-801-88221-4.
75. US history.org, Ancient civilisations, prehistoric times.
76. Brunet et al. A new hominid from the Upper Miocene of Chad, Central Africa, Nature; 2002; 418, 145-151. http://dx.doi.org/10.1038/nature00879
77. Cosgrove, KP; Mazure CM; Staley JK. "Evolving Knowledge of Sex Differences in Brain Structure, Function and Chemistry". Biol Psychiat; 2007; 62 (8): 847–55. doi:10.1016/j.biopsych.2007.03.001. PMC 2711771. PMID 17544382.
78. Swisher, Carl Celso III; Curtis, Garniss H. and Lewin, Roger, Java Man, Abacus, (2002) ISBN 0-349-11473-0.

79. Ruhlen, Merritt. The origin of language: tracing the evolution of the mother tongue. New York: Wiley. (1994) ISBN 0-471-58426-6.
80. Billings, Tom. Humanity's Evolutionary Prehistoric Diet and Ape Diets--continued, Part D. Retrieved 2014-07-11.
81. Grine FE. Dental evidence for dietary differences in Australopithecus and Paranthropus - a quantitative-analysis of permanent molar microwear. Journal of Human Evolution; 1986; 15 (8): 783–822. doi: 10.1016/S0047-2484(86)80010-0.
82. The Ancient Levant, UCL Institute of Archaeology, May 2008
83. Egyptian Journal of Geology - Volume 42, Issue 1 - Page 263, 1998
84. Discover Magazine; 1993; The Naked and the Bipedal
85. Nestle M. Animal vs plant foods in human diets and health: is the historical record unequivocal? Proc. Nutr. Soc; 1999; 58: 211-218.
86. Neil T. Roach, Madhusudhan Venkadesan, Michael J. Rainbow & Daniel E. Lieberman. Elastic energy storage in the shoulder and the evolution of high-speed throwing in Homo Nature; 2013; 498, 483–486 doi:10.1038/nature12267
87. William H. Calvin. A brief history of the mind: From apes to intellect and beyond (2005)
88. William H. Calvin. The Evolution of Human Minds. (20.8.2007)
89. Bilsborough, S.; Mann, N. A review of issues of dietary protein intake in humans. International Journal of Sport Nutrition and Exercise Metabolism; 2006;16, 2, 129–152. PMID 16779921
90. Vilhjalmur Stefansson. Rabbit Starvation, high protein and high fat diets. (1927)
91. John D. Speth; The Paleoanthropology and Archaeology of Big-Game Hunting: Protein, Fat, or Politics? (2012)
92. Ledger, H.P. Body composition as a basis for a comparative study of some East African mammals. Symp. Zool. Soc. London; 1968; 21, 289–310.
93. Richard Francis Burton, The Lake Regions of Central Africa, A Picture of Exploration, (1860)
94. Wrangham, Richard; Conklin-Brittain, NancyLou. Cooking as a biological trait. Comparative Biochemistry and Physiology - Part A: Molecular & Integrative Physiology; 2003;136 (1): 35–46. doi:10.1016/S1095-6433(03)00020-5. PMID 14527628.
95. Marlowe, F. W. The Hadza: Hunter-Gatherers of Tanzania. Berkeley: Univ. California (2010) Press. ISBN 978-0-520-25342-1

References

96. Lee, Richard B. The Cambridge Encyclopedia of Hunters and Gatherers. Daly, Richard Heywood. Cambridge University Press. (1999) ISBN 0-521-57109-X.
97. Hadza people - wikipedia: en.wikipedia.org/wiki/Hadza_people
98. Crittenden, A.N. The Importance of Honey Consumption in Human Evolution (pdf). Food and Foodways; 2011; 19: 257–273. doi: 10.1080/07409710.2011.630618.
99. John D. Speth; Bison Kills and Bone Counts: Decision Making by Ancient Hunters (Prehistoric Archeology and Ecology) (1983)
100. Milton, K. A hypothesis to explain the role of meat-eating in human evolution. Evolutionary Anthropology; 1999; 8, 11-2.
101. Andrews, P. & Martin, L. Hominoid dietary evolution. Philosophical Transactions of the Royal Society of London B 334, 199-209 (1991).
102. Graves RR, Lupo AC, McCarthy RC, Wescott DJ, Cunningham DL, Just how strapping was KNM-WT 15000?. J Hum Evol; 2010; 59 (5): 542–554. doi:10.1016/j.jhevol.2010.06.007. PMID 20846707.
103. Aiello, L. C., & Wheeler, P. The Expensive-Tissue Hypothesis: The Brain and the Digestive System in Human and Primate Evolution. Current Anthropology. 1995; 36(2), 199. doi: 10.1086/204350.
104. Perry GH, Dominy NJ, Claw KG, Lee AS, Fiegler H, Redon R, Werner J, Villanea FA, Mountain JL, Misra R, Carter NP, Lee C, Stone AC. Diet and the evolution of human amylase gene copy number variation. Nature Genetics; 2007;39: 1256-1260.
105. Perry GH, et al. Diet and evolution of human amylase gene copy number variation. Nature Genetics; 2007; 39 (10): 1256–60. doi: 10.1038/ng2123. PMC 2377015. PMID 17828263.
106. Haenel H. Phylogenesis and nutrition. Nahrung 1989; 33 (9): 867–87. PMID 2697806.
107. William H. Calvin. The Evolution of Human Minds. (2007)
108. Board on Science and Technology for International Development, Office of International Affairs, Policy and Global Affairs, National Research Council. Lost Crops of Africa: Volume I: Grains. Washington, DC: The National Academies Press (1996) ISBN: 978-0-309-04990-0
109. Noel D. Vietmeyer, study director of Lost Crops of Africa
110. Trypsin inhibitor, Wikipedia: en.wikipedia.org/wiki/Trypsin_inhibitor
111. Mat Chaudhry Green Gold: Value-added pulses Quantum Media. (2011) ISBN 1-61364-696-8
112. Legume, Wikipedia
113. Pulses: The Perfect Food Developed for the Northern Pulse Growers Association by Julie Garden-Robinson, Ph.D., L.R.D., Food and

References

Nutrition Specialist, North Dakota State University Extension Service. (2012)
114. Beaninstitute.com. August 13, 2013. Retrieved December 17, 2014.
115. MacLarnon AM. The vertebrate canal. In Walker A, Leakey R. The Nariokotome Homo erectus Skeleton. Harvard University Press. (1993) pp. 359–390. ISBN 9780674600751.
116. MacLarnon AM, Hewitt GP. The evolution of human speech: the role of enhanced breathing control. Am J Phys Anthropol;1999; 109(3):341-63. PMID 10407464
117. Gray, Peter B. The Evolution and Endocrinology of Human Behavior: a Focus on Sex Differences and Reproduction. Cambridge, UK: Cambridge University Press. (2010) pp. 277–292. ISBN 978-0-521-70510-3.
118. Gibbons, Ann. Paleoanthropology: Ancient Island Tools Suggest Homo erectus Was a Seafarer. Science; 1998; 279 (5357): 1635–1637. doi: 10.1126/science.279.5357.1635.
119. Marlowe, F. W.. Hunter-gatherers and human evolution. Evolutionary Anthropology: Issues, News, and Reviews; 2005; 14 (2): 54–67. doi: 10.1002/evan.20046.
120. Lee, Richard B. Cambridge Encyclopedia of Hunters and Gatherers. Cambridge University Press. (2005) inside front cover. ISBN 9780521609197.
121. Binford, Louis. R. Human ancestors: Changing views of their behavior. Journal of Anthropological Archaeology; 1986; 3:235-257
122. The Last Rain Forests: A World Conservation Atlas by David Attenborough, Mark Collins
123. Greg Laden , Richard Wrangham; Journal of Human Evolution, Volume 49, Issue 4, October 2005, Pages 482–498; The rise of the hominids as an adaptive shift in fallback foods: Plant underground storage organs (USOs) and australopith origins.
124. Kaplan, H., Hill, K., Lancaster, J. and Hurtado, A. M. A theory of human life history evolution: Diet, intelligence, and longevity. Evol. Anthropol; 2000; 9: 156–185. doi: 10.1002/1520-6505(2000)9:4<156::AID-EVAN5>3.0.CO;2-7
125. Benditt, John. Cold water on the fire: a recent survey casts doubt on evidence for early use of fire. Scientific American; 1989; pp. 21-22.
126. Megarry, Tim. Society in Prehistory: The Origins of Human Culture. New York: New York University Press. (1995)
127. Stranahan AM, Lee K, Martin B, et al. Voluntary exercise and caloric restriction enhance hippocampal dendritic spine density and BDNF

References

levels in diabetic mice. Hippocampus; 2009;19,10, 951-961. doi: 10.1002/hipo.20577.
128. Swisher, Carl Celso III; Curtis, Garniss H. and Lewin, Roger, Java Man, Abacus, (2002) ISBN 0-349-11473-0.
129. Walker, Alan; Shipman, Pat . The Wisdom of Bones : In Search of Human Origins. Weidenfeld and Nicholson, London, 1996, page 240
130. Smithsonian Institution National Museum of American History. "Ancient DNA and Neanderthals". si.edu.
131. Eran Meshorer, Liran Carmel, et al. Reconstructing the DNA Methylation Maps of the Neandertal and the Denisovan. Science; 2014; doi:10.1126/science.1250368.
132. Reid GBR, Hetherington R. The climate connection: climate change and modern human evolution. Cambridge, UK: Cambridge University Press. (2010) p. 64. ISBN 0-521-14723-9.
133. Whitfield, John. Lovers not fighters. Scientific American. (2008)
134. Moskvitch, Katia. Neanderthals were able to 'develop their own tools'. BBC News (BBC). (2010-09-24) Retrieved 2014-11-11.
135. Wilford, John Noble. Neanderthals and the Dead. New York Times. (December 16, 2013) Retrieved December 23, 2014.
136. Roebroeks W, Villa P. On the earliest evidence for habitual use of fire in Europe. Proc Natl Acad Sci. 2011; 108: 5209–5214. doi: 10.1073/pnas.1018116108
137. Dennis M. Sandgathea,b,1, Harold L. Dibblec,d,e, Paul Goldbergf,g, Shannon P. McPherrond, Alain Turqh, Laura Nivend, and Jamie Hodgkinse. Timing of the appearance of habitual fire use. PNAS; 2011;108, 29
138. James, Steven R.. Hominid Use of Fire in the Lower and Middle Pleistocene: A Review of the Evidence. Current Anthropology (University of Chicago Press); 1989; 30 (1): 1–26. doi:10.1086/203705. Retrieved 2012-04-04.
139. Wrangham R. Catching fire: How cooking made us human. New York: Basic Books; 2009.
140. Karen Hardy, Stephen Buckley, Matthew J. Collins, Almudena Estalrrich, Don Brothwell, Les Copeland, Antonio García-Tabernero, Samuel García-Vargas, Marco de la Rasilla, Carles Lalueza-Fox, Rosa Huguet, Markus Bastir, David Santamaría, Marco Madella, Julie Wilson, Ángel Fernández Cortés, Antonio Rosas . Neanderthal medics? Evidence for food, cooking, and medicinal plants entrapped in dental calculus. Naturwissenschaften; 2012; 99, 8 , pp 617-626 DOI 10.1007/s00114-012-0942-0

References

141. Amanda G. Henry, Alison S. Brooks, and Dolores R. Piperno; Microfossils in calculus demonstrate consumption of plants and cooked foods in Neanderthal diets (Shanidar III, Iraq; Spy I and II, Belgium). PNAS; 2010; 108 , 2, 486–491, doi: 10.1073/pnas.1016868108 http://www.pnas.org/content/108/2/486.full
142. Amanda G. Henry; Recovering Dietary Information from Extant and Extinct Primates Using Plant Microremains. Int J Primatol; 2012; 33:702–715
143. d
144. Webb, Jonathan. "Oldest human faeces show Neanderthals ate vegetables". BBC News. (25 June 2014)
145. Neanderthals beat modern humans to the seas by 50,000 years, say scientists".
146. Charles Choi."Ancient Mariners: Did Neanderthals Sail to Mediterranean?". http://www.livescience.com/24810-neanderthals-sailed-mediterranean.html
147. Qiaomei Fu, Heng Li, Priya Moorjani, Flora Jay, Sergey M. Slepchenko, Aleksei A. Bondarev, Philip L. F. Johnson, Ayinuer Aximu-Petri, Kay Prüfer, Cesare de Filippo, Matthias Meyer, Nicolas Zwyns, Domingo C. Salazar-García, Yaroslav V. Kuzmin, Susan G. Keates, Pavel A. Kosintsev, Dmitry I. Razhev, Michael P. Richards, Nikolai V. Peristov, Michael Lachmann, Katerina Douka, Thomas F. G. Higham, Montgomery Slatkin, Jean-Jacques Hublin, David Reich et al. Genome sequence of a 45,000-year-old modern human from western Siberia. 2014; Nature 514, 445–449
148. McDougall, Ian; Brown, Francis H.; Fleagle, John G. "Fossil Reanalysis Pushes Back Origin of Homo sapiens". Scientific American; 2005. "Stratigraphic placement and age of modern humans from Kibish, Ethiopia". Nature 433 (7027): 733–736. Bibcode:2005Natur.433..733M. doi:10.1038/nature03258. PMID 15716951. H. sapiens idaltu is a confirmed subspecies, based on 3 craniums dated 0.16 – 0.15 Mya found in Ethiopia (1997/2003)
149. McDougall I, Brown FH, Fleagle, JG. Stratigraphic placement and age of modern humans from Kibish, Ethiopia. Nature; 2005; 433 (7027): 733–736. Bibcode:2005Natur.433..733M. doi:10.1038/nature03258. PMID 15716951.
150. Stringer, C.B. "Evolution of Early Humans". In Steve Jones, Robert Martin, David Pilbeam. The Cambridge Encyclopedia of Human Evolution. Cambridge: Cambridge University Press. p. 242 (1994). ISBN 978-0-521-32370-3. Also ISBN 978-0-521-46786-5

References

151. Alan G. Morris, Anja Heinze, Eva K.F. Chan, Andrew B. Smith, and Vanessa M. Hayes. First Ancient Mitochondrial Human Genome from a Pre-Pastoralist Southern African; Genome Biology and Evolution Advance Access; 2014; doi:10.1093/gbe/evu202
152. George Ferentinos, , Maria Gkioni , Maria Geraga , George Papatheodoro. Early seafaring activity in the southern Ionian Islands, Mediterranean Sea. Journal of Archaeological Scienc 2011,39, 7, 2167–2176 doi:10.1016/j.jas.2012.01.032
153. Cann RL, Stoneking M, Wilson AC. Mitochondrial DNA and human evolution. Nature; 1987; 325 (6099): 31–6. Bibcode:1987Natur. 325...31C. doi:10.1038/325031a0. PMID 3025745.
154. Vigilant L, Stoneking M, Harpending H, Hawkes K, Wilson AC. African populations and the evolution of human mitochondrial DNA. Science; 1991; 253 (5027): 1503–7.
155. Dawkins, Richard, The Grasshopper's Tale, The Ancestor's Tale, A Pilgrimage to the Dawn of Life, Boston: Houghton Mifflin Company, (2004) p. 416, ISBN 0-297-82503-8, ISBN
156. Jones, Marie; John Savino. Supervolcano: The Catastrophic Event That Changed the Course of Human History (Could Yellowstone be Next?). Franklin Lakes, NJ: New Page Books. (2007) ISBN 1-56414-953-6.
157. http://www.sciencemuseum.org.uk/WhoAmI/FindOutMore/Yourbrain/
158. Quentin D. Atkinson. Phonemic Diversity Supports a Serial Founder Effect Model of Language Expansion from Africa. Science; 2011; 332, 6027, 346-349 DOI: 10.1126/science.1199295
159. Wolfgang Enard, Molly Przeworski, Simon E. Fisher, Cecilia S. L. Lai, Victor Wiebe, Takashi Kitano, Anthony P. Monaco & Svante Pääbo; Molecular evolution of FOXP2, a gene involved in speech and language. Nature; 2005; 418, 869-872
160. Human Natures: Genes, Cultures, and the Human Prospect. Island Press. pp. 159–160. (2002) ISBN 978-1-55963-779-4.
161. WW Norton. Guns, Germs, and Steel: The Fate of Human Societies. W. W. Norton. p. 39. (1999) ISBN 978-0-393-31755-8.
162. Sally Mcbrearty, Alison S. Brooks. The revolution that wasn't: a new interpretation of the origin of modern human behavior. Journal of Human Evolution; 2000; 39, 453–563 doi:10.1006/jhev.2000.0435
163. Jones, Marie; John Savino. Supervolcano: The Catastrophic Event That Changed the Course of Human History (Could Yellowstone be Next?). Franklin Lakes, NJ: New Page Books. (2007) ISBN 1-56414-953-6.

References

164. Self, Stephen; Blake, Stephen. Consequences of Explosive Supereruptions. Elements; 2008; 4 (1): 41–46. doi:10.2113/GSELEMENTS.4.1.41.
165. Zielinski, G. A.; Mayewski, P. A.; Meeker, L.D.; Whitlow, S.; Twickler, M.S.; Taylor, K. (1996). Potential Atmospheric Impact of the Toba Mega-Eruption ~71,000 years ago. Geophysical Research Letters; 2008; 23 (8): 837–840. Bibcode:1996GeoRL..23..837Z. doi: 10.1029/96GL00706.
166. Takahata N, Allelic genealogy and human evolution, Mol Biol Evol; 1993; 10 (1): 2–22, PMID 8450756.
167. Schaffner, SF, The X chromosome in population genetics, Nat Rev Genet; 2004; 5 (1): 43–51, doi:10.1038/nrg1247, PMID 14708015
168. Reid GBR, Hetherington R. The climate connection: climate change and modern human evolution. Cambridge, UK: Cambridge University Press. (2010) p. 64. ISBN 0-521-14723-9.
169. Kennedy, Kenneth Adrian Raine. God-Apes and Fossil Men: Palaeoanthropology of South Asia. Ann Arbor: University of Michigan Press. (2000)
170. John N Wilford. Fossil Teeth Put Humans in Europe Earlier Than Thought. The New York Times. 2011-11-02.
171. McHenry, H.M. Human Evolution. In Michael Ruse & Joseph Travis. Evolution: the first four billion years. Cambridge, Massachusetts: The Belknap Press of Harvard University Press. p. 265. (2009) ISBN 978-0-674-03175-3.
172. Nicholas Wade. "Before the Dawn" (2007) ISBN-13: 978-0143038320
173. Prehistoric Archaeological Periods in Japan, Charles T. Keally
174. World Museum of Man: Neolithic / Chalcolithic Period". World Museum of Man. Retrieved 22 October 2014.
175. Kislev, Mordechai E, Hartmann Anat & Bar-Yosef, Ofer. Early Domesticated Fig in the Jordan Valley. Science; 2006a; 312(5778): 1372. doi:10.1126/science.1125910 PMID 16741119 (HTML abstract) Supporting Online Material
176. The Development of Agriculture". National Geographic. Retrieved 27 December 2014.
177. Jared Diamond. Once upon a time, all the fruits, nuts, and berries our gathering ancestors ate were wild. Someone, at some time, had to come up with the bright idea of crops. Discovery Magazine - Biology and Medicine; September 1994.
178. Roberts, J. History of the World. Penguin (1996)

References

179. Cunliffe, Barry. Prehistoric Europe: an Illustrated History. Oxford University Press; (1998)
180. The Bradshaw Foundation: www.bradshawfoundation.com/journey/agriculture2.html
181. McNeilage A. Diet and habitat use of two mountain gorilla groups in contrasting habitats in the Virungas. In: Robbins MM, Sicotte P, Stewart KJ, editors. Mountain gorillas: three decades of research at Karisoke. Cambridge (England): Cambridge University Press. pp. 265–92. (2001)
182. Calvert, J. Food selection by western gorillas (G. g. gorilla) in relation to food chemistry. Oecologia; 1985; 65, 2, 236-246
183. Tutin C.E.G., Fernandez M. Composition of the diet of chimpanzees and comparisons with that of sympatric lowland gorillas in the Lopé Reserve, Gabon. Am. J. Primatol; 1993; 30:195–211
184. 2014 SeaWorld Parks & Entertainment Gorilla Diet and eating Habits
185. Yamagiwa J, Mwanza N, Yumoto T, Maruhashi T. "Seasonal change in the composition of the diet of eastern lowland gorillas". Primates; 1994; 35: 1.
186. Williamson EA, Tutin CE, Rogers ME, Fernandez M. Composition of the diet of lowland gorillas at Lope in Gabon. Am J Primatol; 1990; 21:265–277
187. Williamson E. Behavioural ecology of western lowland gorillas in Gabon. University of Stirling, Stirling (1988)
188. Rogers E, Williamson E Density of herbaceous plants eaten by gorillas in Gabon: some preliminary data. Biotropica; 1987; 19:278–281
189. Casimir, M.J. Feeding ecology and nutrition of an eastern gorilla group in the Mt. Kahuzi region (Republic of Zaire). Folia Primatologica; 1975; 24:81-136.
190. Kleiber M. "Body size and metabolic rate". Physiological Reviews; 1947; 27 ,4, 511–541. PMID 20267758.
191. Food and nutrition technical report series. Human energy requirements. Report of a Joint FAO/WHO/UNU Expert Consultation. (October 2001)
192. Mahaney, W.C., D.P. Watts, and R.G.V. Hancock. Geophagia by mountain gorillas (Gorilla gorilla beringei) in the Virunga mountains, Rwanda. Primates; 1990; 31:113-120.
193. Ammerman, C.B., D.H. Baker, and A.J. Lewis, Eds. Bioavailability of Nutrients for Animals. San Diego: Academic Press. (1995)
194. Institute of Medicine (US) & Institute of Medicine (US), 2005; Lissner et al., 1987; USHSS, 2010; WHO, 2003

References

195. Bjerve K, Mostad I, Thoresen L. Alpha-linolenic acid deficiency in patients on long-term gastric tube feeding; estimation of linolenic acid and long chain unsaturated n-3 fatty acid requirements in man. Am J Clin Nutr; 1987; 45:66–77.
196. Holman RT. The slow discovery of the importance of omega 3 essential fatty acids in human health. J Nutr; 1998; 128:427S–433S.
197. Moriguchi T, Salem N Jr. Recovery of brain docosahex- aenoate leads to recovery of spatial task performance. J Neurochem; 2003; 87:297–309.
198. Uauy R, Dangour AD. Nutrition in brain development and aging: role of essential fatty acids. Nutr Rev; 2006; 64:S24– S33.
199. Brenna JT, Salem N Jr, Sinclair AJ, Cunnane SC. a-Linolenic acid supplementation and conversion to n-3 long-chain polyunsaturated fatty acids in humans. Prosta- glandins Leukot Essent Fatty Acids; 2009; 80:85–91.
200. Su H-M, Corso TN, Nathanielsz PW, Brenna TJ. Linoleic acid kinetics and conversion to arachidonic acid in the pregnant and fetal baboon. J Lipid Res; 1999; 40:1304–1311.
201. M. Henneberg. Secular trends in body height - indicator of general improvement in living conditions or of a change in specific factors. Perspectives in Human Growth, Development and Maturation. Parasmani Dasgupta, Roland Hauspie. Springer Science & Business Media; 2001; 14, 159-167.
202. Andrews, P. & Martin, L. Hominoid dietary evolution. Philosophical Transactions of the Royal Society of London B 334, 199-209 (1991).
203. Milton, K. A hypothesis to explain the role of meat-eating in human evolution. Evolutionary Anthropology; 1999; 8, 11-2.
204. Jolly, C. J. The seed-eaters: a new model of hominid differentiation based on a baboon analogy. Man; 1970; 5, 1-26.
205. Peters, C. R., O'Brian, E. M. The early hominid plant-food niche: insights from an analysis of plant exploitation by Homo, Pan, and Papio in eastern and southern Africa. Current Anthropology; 1981; 22, 127-140
206. Teaford, M. F. & Ungar, P. S. Diet and the evolution of the earliest human ancestors. Proceedings of the National Academy of Sciences; 2000; USA 97, 13506-13511.
207. Jared Diamond, The Worst Mistake in the History of the Human Race, Discover Magazine; 1987; pp. 64-66.

References

208. John Hawks. Selection for smaller brains in Holocene human evolution. John Hawks webblog. Department of Anthropology University of Wisconsin (2011)
209. Cohen MN, Armelagos GJ. Paleopathology and the Origins of Agriculture London: Academic Press. (1984)
210. Milton K, et al. The role of food processing factors in primate food choice" Primate feeding ecology; P roman and J Cant, eds. New York: Columbia. U press. 1979; 249-279
211. Hazarika, Manji. Homo erectus/ergaster and Out of Africa: Recent Developments in Paleoanthropology and Prehistoric Archaeology. Universitat Rovira i Virgili, Tarragona, Spain; EAA Summer School eBook; 2007; 1: 35-41
212. Peter Bellwood. The Origins of Agricultural Societies (2004)
213. Historical Estimates of World Population. US Census Bureau. Archived from the original on 2 January 2011. Retrieved 16 October December 2014
214. Bocquet-Appel JP: When the World's Population Took Off: The Springboard of the Neolithic Demographic Transition. Science; 2011; 333 (6042) : 560-561.
215. Jared Diamond. Once upon a time, all the fruits, nuts, and berries our gathering ancestors ate were wild. Someone, at some time, had to come up with the bright idea of crops. Discovery Magazine - Biology and Medicine; September 1994.
216. ipm.ncsu.edu Pesticide and fertilizer use: ipm.ncsu.edu/safety/factsheets/pestuse.pdf
217. American Museum of Natural History: www.amnh.org/exhibitions/past-exhibitions/horse/domesticating-horses/domestication-timeline
218. Ann Gibbons. The Evolution of Diet. National Geographic Magazine (2013)
219. K. Klein Goldewijk and G. van Drecht. "HYDE 3.1: Current and historical population and land cover"., Data from History Database of the Global Environment. (2007)
220. Colin McEvedy and Richard Jones. Atlas of World Population History, Facts on File, New York,(1978) ISBN 0-7139-1031-3.
221. World Population Meter: www.worldometers.info/world-population/
222. United Nations, Department of Economic and Social Affairs, Population Division (2013). World Population Prospects: The 2012 Revision, Press Release (13 June 2013): "World Population to reach 9.6 billion by 2050 with most growth in developing regions, especially Africa".

References

223. Board on Science and Technology for International Development, Office of International Affairs, Policy and Global Affairs, National Research Council. Lost Crops of Africa: Volume I: Grains. Washington, DC: The National Academies Press (1996) ISBN: 978-0-309-04990-0
224. Eaton SB, Konner M. Paleolithic nutrition: a consideration of its nature and current implications. New Engl. J. Med; 1985; 312: 283-289.
225. Cordain L. Cereal grains: humanity's double-edged sword. Wld Rev. Nutr. Diet; 1999; 84: 19-73.
226. Eades MR, Eades MD. The Protein Power Lifeplan New York: Warner Books. (2000)
227. Worm N. Syndrom X oder ein Mammut auf den Teller. Mit Steinzeit-Diät aus det Wohl stands Falle. Systemed-Verlag, Lünen. (2002).
228. Cohen MN, Armelagos GJ. Paleopathology and the Origins of Agriculture London: Academic Press. (1984)
229. M P Richards; A brief review of the archaeological evidence for Palaeolithic and Neolithic subsistence; European Journal of Clinical Nutrition; 2002; 56, 12, 1270-1278
230. Rolland Nicolas. Was the emergence of home bases and domestic fire a punctuated event? A review of the Middle Pleistocene record in Eurasia. Asian Perspectives: the Journal of Archaeology for Asia and the Pacific; 2004; 43, 248-281.
231. Hillard Kaplan, Kim Hill, Jane Lancaster, and A. Magdalena Hurtado. "A Theory of Human Life History Evolution: Diet, Intelligence and Longevity". Evolutionary Anthropology ;2000; 9 (4): 156–185. doi: 10.1002/1520-6505(2000)9:4<156::AID-EVAN5>3.0.CO;2-7.
232. Kramer, K.L. & Greaves, R.D.. Changing patterns of infant mortality and maternal fertility among Pume foragers and horticulturalists. American Anthropologist; 2007; 109(4), 713-726.
233. Leaky MD, Hay RL. Pliocene footprints in the Laetolil Beds at laetoli, northern Tanzania. Nature; 1979; 278:317-323
234. Hewlett, B.S.. Demography and childcare in preindustrial societies. Journal of Anthropological Research; 1991; 47(1), 1-37.
235. United Nations, Department of Economic and Social Affairs, Population Division. World Population Prospects: The 2012 Revision, (2013).
236. Tony Volk, Jeremy Atkinson. Is Child Death The Crucible Of Human Evolution? Journal of Social, Evolutionary, and Cultural Psychology; Proceedings of the 2nd Annual Meeting of the NorthEastern Evolutionary Psychology Society (2008)

References

237. Galor, O, Moav, O. "The Neolithic Revolution and Contemporary Variations in Life Expectancy". Brown University Working Paper. (2007)
238. Thomson Prentice. Health, history and hard choices: Funding dilemmas in a fast-changing world. Global Health Histories, WHO, Health and Philanthropy: Leveraging change University of Indiana, (2006)
239. United Nations, Department of Economic and Social Affairs, Population Division. World Population Prospects: The 2012 Revision, (2013).
240. Miniño AM, Murphy SL, Xu JQ, Kochanek KD. Deaths: Final data for 2008. National vital statistics reports; vol 59 no 10. Hyattsville, MD: National Center for Health Statistics. 2011. Available from: http://www.cdc.gov/nchs/data/nvsr/nvsr59/nvsr59_10.pdf.
241. Kochanek KD, Martin JA. Supplemental analyses of recent trends in infant mortality. Health E-Stat. Hyattsville, MD: National Center for Health Statistics. Available from: http://www.cdc.gov/nchs/data/hestat/infantmort/infantmort.htm.
242. Donna L. Hoyert, Jiaquan Xu. National Vital, Statistics Reports, Volume 61, Number 6; Deaths: Preliminary Data for 2011; Division of Vital Statistics (2012)
243. AHA Statistical Update. Heart Disease and Stroke Statistics—2015 Update. A Report From the American Heart Association. Circulation; 2015; 131: e29-e322. doi: 10.1161/CIR.0000000000000152
244. Chronic Care in America: A 21st Century Challenge, a study of the Robert Wood Johnson Foundation & Partnership for Solutions: Johns Hopkins University, Baltimore, MD for the Robert Wood Johnson Foundation (September 2004 Update). "Chronic Conditions: Making the Case for Ongoing Care".
245. Thomson Prentice. Health, history and hard choices: Funding dilemmas in a fast-changing world. Global Health Histories, WHO, Health and Philanthropy: Leveraging change University of Indiana, (2006)
246. Gerard Anderson. The Growing Burden of Chronic Disease in American, Public Health Reports; 2004,119
247. National Public Radio - news & analysis: www.npr.org/templates/search/index.php?searchinput=meat+consumption
248. AHA Statistical Update. Heart Disease and Stroke Statistics—2015 Update. A Report From the American Heart Association. Circulation; 2015; 131: e29-e322. doi: 10.1161/CIR.0000000000000152

References

249. Wikipedia, Agriculture: en.wikipedia.org/wiki/Agricultur
250. Wessel, T.. "The Agricultural Foundations of Civilization". Journal of Agriculture and Human Values; 1984; 1:9–12
251. Eaton SB, Konner M, Shostak M. Stone agers in the fast lane: Chronic degenrative diseases in evolutionary perspective; Am J Med; 1988:84;739-749.
252. Simopolous AP. Is insulin resistance influenced by dietary linoleum acid and trans fatty acids? Free Rad Biol Med; 1994;17:367-372.
253. Horton ES. Exercise and decreased risk of NIDDM. N Engl J Med; 1991;325:196-198.
254. DK Jordan. Living the Revolution. The Neolithic. University of California – San Diego. (2012) Retrieved 22 September 2014.
255. Finlay, B. L. & Darlington, R. B. Linked regularities in the development and evolution of mammalian brains. Science; 1995; 268: 1578-1584.
256. Lee, R. B. What hunters do for a living, in Man The Hunter, (1968) pp. 38-48
257. Peters C. R. and O'brien E. M. The early hominid plant food niche: Insights from an analysis of plant exploitation by Homo, Pan, Papio in eastern and southern Africa, Current Anthropology; 1981; 22:127-140.
258. Henry AG, Brooks AS, Piperno DR, Microfossils in calculus demonstrate consumption of plants and cooked foods in Neanderthal diets (Shanidar III, Iraq; Spy I and II, Belgium); Proc Natl Acad Sci U S A; 2011; 11;108(2):486-91. doi: 10.1073/pnas.1016868108. Epub 2010 Dec 27.
259. Henry AG, Brooks AS, Piperno DR; Plant foods and the dietary ecology of Neanderthals and early modern humans. J Hum Evol; 2014; Apr; 69:44-54. doi: 10.1016/j.jhevol.2013.12.014. Epub 2014 Mar 5.
260. Lee, R. B.what hunters do for a living in Man The Hunter (1968), pp. 38-48
261. Woodburn. J. C. An introduction to Hadza ecology. In Man the hunter (eds) R. B. Lee &. I. DeVore. Chicago: Aldlne. (1968)
262. Clifford J. Jolly. The Seed-Eaters: A New Model of Hominid Differentiation Based on a Baboon Analogy. Man; 1970; 5, 1, 5-26.
263. Peters C. R. and O'brien E. M. The early hominin plant food niche: Insights from an analysis of plant exploitation by Homo, Pan, Papio in eastern and southern Africa, Current Anthropology; 1981; 22:127-140.
264. Zilhan A. L. Women in Evolution, II. Subsistence and social organisation among early hominids; 1978; 4(1)
265. Board on Science and Technology for International Development, Office of International Affairs, Policy and Global Affairs, National

References

Research Council. Lost Crops of Africa: Volume I: Grains. Washington, DC: The National Academies Press (1996) ISBN: 978-0-309-04990-0

266. Williams, Cicely. Kwashiorkor. The Lancet; 1935; 226 (5855): 1151. doi: 10.1016/S0140-6736(00)94666-X.

267. Krebs NF, Primak LE, Hambridge KM. Normal childhood nutrition & its disorders. In: Current Pediatric Diagnosis & Treatment. New York: McGraw-Hill; 2003; 17, p. 291-2

268. Youngman LD. The growth and development of aflatoxin B1-induced preneoplastic lesions, tumors, metastasis, and spontaneous tumors as they are influenced by dietary protein level, type, and intervention. Ithaca, NY: Cornell University, Ph.D. Thesis, 1990.

269. Stahl A.B. Hominid dietary selection before fire. current anthropology; 1984; vol. 25, no. 2

270. Watts, D. P. Scavenging by chimpanzees at Ngogo and the relevance of chimpanzee scavenging to early hominin behavioral ecology. Journal of Human Evolution; 2008; 54, 125-133.

271. Ragir, S. et al. Gut morphology and the avoidance of carrion among chimpanzees, baboons, and early hominids. Journal of Anthropological Research; 2000; 56, 477-512.

272. Donald P, Pitts CC, Pohl SL. Body weight and composition in laboratory rats: effects of diets with high or low protein concentrations. Science; 1981;211(4478),185-6.

273. Rothwell NJ, Stock MJ, Tyzbir RS. Mechanisms of thermogenesis induced by low protein diets. Metabolism; 1983;32,3, 257-61.

274. Rothwell NJ, Stock MJ. Influence of carbohydrate and fat intake on diet-induced thermogenesis and brown fat activity in rats fed low protein diets. J Nutr; 1987;117,10,1721-6.

275. Stillings BR. "World supplies of animal protein." In: J. W. G. Porter and B. A. Rolls (eds.), Proteins in Human Nutrition, pp. 11–33. London: Academic Press, (1973).

276. U.S. Department of Agriculture, Agricultural Research Service. 2004. USDA National Nutrient Database for Standard Reference, Release 17. Nutrient Data Laboratory Home Page, http://www.ars.usda.gov/main/site_main.htm?modecode=80-40-05-25.

277. Osthoff G1, Hugo A, de Wit M. The composition of cheetah (Acinonyx jubatus) milk.; Comp Biochem Physiol B Biochem Mol Biol; 2006;145(3-4):265-9.

278. Case Western Reserve University; Gorillas go green: Apes shed pounds while doubling calories on leafy diet, researcher finds; Science Daily (2011)

References

279. University of California - Irvine. Heart disease found in Egyptian mummies. Sciencedaily (2009)
280. Roger Horowitz; Putting Meat on the American Table: Taste, Technology, Transformation; (2006).
281. Esselstyn CB Jr, Ellis SG, Medendorp SV, Crowe TD; A strategy to arrest and reverse coronary artery disease: a 5-year longitudinal study of a single physician's practice. J Fam Pract; 1995; 41(6):560-8.
282. Giuseppe Grosso, Fabio Galvano, Stefano Marventano, et al. Omega-3 Fatty Acids and Depression: Scientific Evidence and Biological Mechanisms. Oxidative Medicine and Cellular Longevity; 2014; 1-16. Article ID 313570; doi:10.1155/2014/313570
283. PM Kris-Etherton, Denise Shaffer Taylor, Shaomei Yu-Poth, Peter Huth, Kristin Moriarty, Valerie Fishell, Rebecca L Hargrove, Guixiang Zhao, and Terry D Etherton. Polyunsaturated fatty acids in the food chain in the United States. Am J Clin Nutr; 2000, 71 ,1, 179S-188S
284. Giuseppe Grosso, Fabio Galvano, Stefano Marventano, et al. Omega-3 Fatty Acids and Depression: Scientific Evidence and Biological Mechanisms. Oxidative Medicine and Cellular Longevity; 2014; 1-16. Article ID 313570; doi:10.1155/2014/313570
285. Goncalves CG, Ramos EJ, Suzuki S, Meguid MM. Omega-3 fatty acids and anorexia. Curr Opin Clin Nutr Metab Care; 2005;8,4,403-7.
286. Omega-3 Fatty Acids as Adjunctive Treatment for Adolescents With Eating Disorders. ClinicalTrials.gov Identifier: NCT01985178 (2013)
287. Simopoulos AP. Omega-3 fatty acids in inflammation and autoimmune diseases. J Am Coll Nutr; 2002;21,6,495-505.
288. Public Health Service's Office in Women's Health, Eating Disorders Information Sheet, (2000).
289. Eric Schlosser. Fast Food Nation: what the all-american meal is doing to the world; Houghton Mifflin Company (2001). ISBN: 978-0-14-194421-0
290. Liu L, Johnson HL, Cousens S, Perin J, Scott S, Lawn JE, Rudan I, Campbell H, Cibulskis R, Li M, Mathers C, Black RE. Child Health Epidemiology Reference Group of WHO and UNICEF. Global, regional, and national causes of child mortality: an updated systematic analysis for 2010 with time trends since 2000. Lancet; 2012;379,9832,2151-61.
291. Centers for Disease Control and Prevention. Data and statistics, Tuberculosis.
292. Felicity Lawrence. The secret of the 'special offer' economy burger. (Jan 2013)

References

293. Agency for Toxic Substances and Disease Registry. Division of Toxicology and Human Health Sciences. Toxic Substances Portal - Ammonia. (retrieved 16 March 2015)
294. Jerry R. Balentine. Sepsis - Blood Infection. eMedicineHealth; 2014.
295. National Center for Health Statistics Data Brief No. 62. Inpatient care for septicemia or sepsis: a challenge for patients and hospitals. (2011)
296. EFSA Panel on Additives and Products or Substances used in Animal Feed (FEEDAP)2,3 European Food Safety Authority (EFSA), Parma, Italy. Scientific Opinion on the safety and efficacy of Maxiban® G160 (narasin and nicarbazin) for chickens for fattening. EFSA Journal; 2010; 8,4,1574
297. Eric Schlosser. Fast Food Nation: what the all-american meal is doing to the world; Houghton Mifflin Company (2001). ISBN: 978-0-14-194421-0
298. "Bovine Spongiform Encephalopaphy: An Overview" (PDF). Animal and Plant Health Inspection Service, United States Department of Agriculture. (2006).
299. Center for Food Safety and Applied Nutrition. "Commonly Asked Questions About BSE in Products Regulated by FDA's Center for Food Safety and Applied Nutrition (CFSAN)". Food and Drug Administration; 2005.
300. Ramasamy, M Law, S Collins, F Brook. Organ distribution of prion proteins in variant Creutzfeldt-Jakob disease. The Lancet Infectious Diseases; 2003; 3 (4): 214–222. doi:10.1016/S1473-3099(03)00578-4. PMID 12679264.
301. Variant Creutzfeld-Jakob Disease, Current Data. The National Creutzfeldt-Jakob Disease Surveillance Unit (NCJDSU), University of Edinburgh. (2009). Retrieved 2014-10-14.
302. Valleron AJ, Boelle PY, Will R, Cesbron JY. Estimation of epidemic size and incubation time based on age characteristics of vCJD in the United Kingdom. Science; 2001; 294 (5547): 1726–8. doi:10.1126/science.1066838. PMID 11721058. Lay summary – BBC News (2001-11-23).
303. W.H. Wilson Tang, Zeneng Wang, Yiying Fan, Bruce Levison, Jennie E. Hazen, Lillian M. Donahue, Yuping Wu, Stanley L. Hazen. Prognostic Value of Elevated Levels of Intestinal Microbe-Generated Metabolite Trimethylamine-N-Oxide in Patients With Heart Failure. Journal of the American College of Cardiology; 2014; 64 (18): 1908 DOI: 10.1016/j.jacc.2014.02.617
304. Pan A, Sun Q, Bernstein AM, et al. Red Meat Consumption and Mortality: Results from Two Prospective Cohort Studies. Archives of

internal medicine; 2012;172(7):555-563. doi:10.1001/archinternmed.2011.2287.
305. Key TJ, Fraser GE, Thorogood M, Appleby PN, Beral V, Reeves G, Burr ML, Chang-Claude J, Frentzel-Beyme R, Kuzma JW, Mann J, McPherson K. Mortality in vegetarians and nonvegetarians: detailed findings from a collaborative analysis of 5 prospective studies. Am J Clin Nutr; 1999; 70(3 Suppl):516S-524S.
306. Aune D, Ursin G, Veierød MB. Meat consumption and the risk of type 2 diabetes: a systematic review and meta-analysis of cohort studies. Diabetologia; 2009;52(11):2277-2287.
307. Pan A, Sun Q, Bernstein AM, et al. Red meat consumption and risk of type 2 diabetes: 3 cohorts of US adults and an updated meta-analysis. Am J Clin Nutr; 2011;94(4):1088-1096.PubMed
308. Pan A, Sun Q, Bernstein AM, Manson JE, Willett WC, Hu FB. Changes in Red Meat Consumption and Subsequent Risk of Type 2 Diabetes Mellitus: Three Cohorts of US Men and Women. JAMA Intern Med; 2013;173(14):1328-1335. doi:10.1001/jamainternmed.2013.6633.
309. Driver, Jane A., Ashley Smith, Julie E. Buring, J. Michael Gaziano, Tobias Kurth, and Giancarlo Logroscino. Prospective cohort study of type 2 diabetes and the risk of Parkinson's disease 2003-2005. Diabetes Care; 2008; 31,10.
310. Bartzokis George, Lu Po H, Tingus Kathleen, Peters Douglas G, Amar Chetan P, Tishler Todd A, Finn J Paul, Villablanca Pablo, Altshuler Lori L, Mintz Jim, Neely Elizabeth, Connor James R Gender and iron genes may modify associations between brain iron and memory in healthy aging Neuropsychopharmacology: official publication of the American College of Neuropsychopharmacology; 2011; 36(7): 1375-84.
311. Raven EP, Lu PO, Tishler TA, Heydari P, Bartzokis G. Increased Iron Levels and Decreased Tissue Integrity in Hippocampus of Alzheimer's Disease Detected in vivo with Magnetic Resonance Imaging. Journal of Alzheimer's Disease; 2013; 37, 127–136 127 DOI 10.3233/JAD-130209 IOS Press
312. Red meat and colon cancer, The Harvard Medical School Family Health Guide (2008)
313. Cho E, Chen WY, Hunter DJ, et al. Red Meat Intake and Risk of Breast Cancer Among Premenopausal Women. Arch Intern Med; 2006;166(20):2253-2259. doi:10.1001/archinte.166.20.2253.
314. Farvid Maryam S, Cho Eunyoung, Chen Wendy Y, Eliassen A Heather, Willett Walter C. Dietary protein sources in early adulthood and breast cancer incidence: prospective cohort study BMJ; 2014; 348, 3437

References

315. Ahmed MK, Shaheen N, Islam MS, Habibullah-Al-Mamun M, Islam S, Mohiduzzaman M, Bhattacharjee L. Dietary intake of trace elements from highly consumed cultured fish (Labeo rohita, Pangasius pangasius and Oreochromis mossambicus) and human health risk implications in Bangladesh.Chemosphere; 2015;128,284-292. doi: 10.1016/j.chemosphere.2015.02.016.
316. Cai LM, Xu ZC, Qi JY, Feng ZZ, Xiang TS. Assessment of exposure to heavy metals and health risks among residents near Tonglushan mine in Hubei, China. Chemosphere; 2015; 127,127-135. doi: 10.1016/j.chemosphere.2015.01.027.
317. Cancer in Animals and Fish: www.earthfuture.com/cancer/files/Cancer_in_Animals.pdf
318. Lukiw WJ, Cui JG, Marcheselli VL, Bodker M, Botkjaer A, Gotlinger K, Serhan CN, Bazan NG.; Cui; Marcheselli; Bodker; Botkjaer; Gotlinger; Serhan; Bazan. "A role for docosahexaenoic acid-derived neuroprotectin D1 in neural cell survival and Alzheimer disease". J Clin Invest; 2005; 115 ,10, 2774–83. doi:10.1172/JCI25420. PMC 1199531. PMID 16151530.
319. Kelley DS et al. DHA supplementation decreases serum C-reactive protein and other markers of inflammation in hypertriglyceridemic men. J Nutr; 2009;139,3,495-501.
320. Pauwels, E. K.; Kostkiewicz, M. Fatty acid facts, Part III: Cardiovascular disease, or, a fish diet is not fishy. Drug news & perspectives; 2008; 21 , 10, 552–61. doi:10.1358/dnp.2008.21.10.1314058 (inactive 2015-02-07). PMID 19221636.
321. Samieri, C; Lorrain, S; Buaud, B; Vaysse, C; Berr, C; Peuchant, E; Cunnane, S. C.; Barberger-Gateau, P. "Relationship between diet and plasma long-chain n-3 PUFAs in older people: Impact of apolipoprotein E genotype". The Journal of Lipid Research; 2013; 54 ,9, 2559–67. doi: 10.1194/jlr.P036475. PMC 3735952. PMID 23801662.
322. Bazan, N. G.; Molina, M. F.; Gordon, W. C.. "Docosahexaenoic acid signalolipidomics in nutrition: Significance in aging, neuroinflammation, macular degeneration, Alzheimer's, and other neurodegenerative diseases". Annual Review of Nutrition; 2011; 31,321–51. doi:10.1146/annurev.nutr.012809.104635. PMC 3406932. PMID 21756134.
323. Bousquet, M; Saint-Pierre, M; Julien, C; Salem Jr, N; Cicchetti, F; Calon, F. Beneficial effects of dietary omega-3 polyunsaturated fatty acid on toxin-induced neuronal degeneration in an animal model of Parkinson's disease. The FASEB Journal; 2008; 22,4, 1213–25. doi: 10.1096/fj.07-9677com. PMID 18032633.

References

324. Kathleen Blanchard. DHA in Fish Oil Could Protect from Stroke Disability. Louisiana State University. (2010)
325. Jakobsen SE, Lie E. "New treatment for psoriasis". ScienceNordic. (2013)
326. Paul Shapiro, vice president of farm animal protection for The HSUS
327. Weaver CM, Heaney R. Calcium, Modern Nutrition in Health and Disease. 10. Shils ME, Shike M, Ross AC, Cabellero B, Cousins RJ, editors. Baltimore, MD: Lippincott Williams & Wilkins; (2006).
328. Escott-Stump S, ed. Nutrition and Diagnosis Related Care. 6th ed. Philadelphia, Pa: Lippincott Williams and Wilkins; (2008).
329. Osteoporosis: A guide to prevention and treatment. Harvard Health Publications, 2010
330. Mélanie Salque, Peter I. Bogucki, Joanna Pyzel, Iwona Sobkowiak-Tabaka, Ryszard Grygiel, Marzena Szmyt, Richard P. Evershed. Earliest evidence for cheese making in the sixth millennium BC in northern Europe; Nature; 2013; 493, 522–525 doi:10.1038/nature11698 http://dx.doi.org/10.1038/nature11698 (2012).
331. Cristina Gamba, Eppie R. Jones, Matthew D. Teasdale, Russell L. McLaughlin, Gloria Gonzalez-Fortes, Valeria Mattiangeli, László Domboróczki, Ivett Kővári, Ildikó Pap, Alexandra Anders, Alasdair Whittle, János Dani, Pál Raczky, Thomas F. G. Higham, Michael Hofreiter, Daniel G. Bradley & Ron Pinhasi; Genome flux and stasis in a five millennium transect of European prehistory; Nature Communications; 2014; 5, (5257) doi:10.1038/ncomms6257.
332. Dunne, J., Evershed, R.P., Cramp, L.J.E., Bruni, S., Biagetti, S. and di Lernia, S. The beginnings of Dairying as practised by Pastoralists in 'Green' Saharan Africa in the 5th Millennium BC. Documenta Praehistorica; 2013; 40, 118-130
333. Dunne, J., Evershed, R.P., Salque, M., Cramp, L., Bruni, S., Ryan, K., Biagetti, S., and di Lernia, S. First dairying in green Saharan Africa in the fifth millennium BC. Nature; 2012; 486, 390-394
334. Cristina Gamba, Eppie R. Jones, Matthew D. Teasdale, Russell L. McLaughlin, Gloria Gonzalez-Fortes, Valeria Mattiangeli, László Domboróczki, Ivett Kővári, Ildikó Pap, Alexandra Anders, Alasdair Whittle, János Dani, Pál Raczky, Thomas F. G. Higham, Michael Hofreiter, Daniel G. Bradley & Ron Pinhasi; Genome flux and stasis in a five millennium transect of European prehistory; Nature Communications; 2014; 5, (5257) doi:10.1038/ncomms6257.
335. Bogucki, P. I. Oxford J. Archaeol; 1984; 3, 15–30.

References

336. Dunne, J., Evershed, R.P., Cramp, L.J.E., Bruni, S., Biagetti, S. and di Lernia, S. The beginnings of Dairying as practised by Pastoralists in 'Green' Saharan Africa in the 5th Millennium BC. Documenta Praehistorica; 2013; 40, 118-130
337. Dunne, J., Evershed, R.P., Salque, M., Cramp, L., Bruni, S., Ryan, K., Biagetti, S., and di Lernia, S. First dairying in green Saharan Africa in the fifth millennium BC. Nature; 2012; 486, 390-394
338. Paul Shapiro, vice president of farm animal protection for The HSUS
339. Institute of Medicine (US) Committee to Review Dietary Reference Intakes for Vitamin D and Calcium; Ross AC, Taylor CL, Yaktine AL, et al., editors. Dietary Reference Intakes for Calcium and Vitamin D. Washington (DC): National Academies Press (US); 2011; 2, Overview of Calcium.
340. Dunne, J., Evershed, R.P., Cramp, L.J.E., Bruni, S., Biagetti, S. and di Lernia, S. The beginnings of Dairying as practised by Pastoralists in 'Green' Saharan Africa in the 5th Millennium BC. Documenta Praehistorica; 2013; 40, 118-130
341. Owusu W, Willett WC, Feskanich D, Ascherio A, Spiegelman D, Colditz GA. Calcium intake and the incidence of forearm and hip fractures among men. J Nutr; 1997; 127:1782–87.
342. Feskanich D, Willett WC, Stampfer MJ, Colditz GA. Milk, dietary calcium, and bone fractures in women: a 12-year prospective study. Am J Public Health; 1997; 87:992–97.
343. Bischoff-Ferrari HA, Dawson-Hughes B, Baron JA, et al. Calcium intake and hip fracture risk in men and women: a meta-analysis of prospective cohort studies and randomized controlled trials. Am J Clin Nutr; 2007; 86:1780–90.
344. Feskanich D, Bischoff-Ferrari HA, Frazier AL, Willett WC. Milk consumption during teenage years and risk of hip fractures in older adults. JAMA Pediatr; 2014;168(1):54-60.
345. Lanou AJ, Berkow SE, Barnard ND. Calcium, dairy products, and bone health in children and young adults: a reevaluation of the evidence. Pediatrics; 2005;115:736–743.
346. Sonneville KR, Gordon CM, Kocher MS, Pierce LM, Ramappa A, Field AE. Vitamin D, calcium, and dairy intakes and stress fractures among female adolescents. Arch Pediatr Adolesc Med; 2012;166:595-600.
347. Calcium and Milk | The Nutrition Source | Harvard School of Public Health hsph.harvard.edu

References

348. Feskanich D, Willett WC, Colditz GA. Calcium, vitamin D, milk consumption, and hip fractures: a prospective study among postmenopausal women. Am J Clin Nutr; 2003;77:504–511.
349. Richard B. Mazess and Warren Mather. Bone mineral content of North Alaskan Eskimos; Am J Clin Nutr ; 1974; 27, 9, 916-925
350. Ioannis Delimaris, "Adverse Effects Associated with Protein Intake above the Recommended Dietary Allowance for Adults," ISRN Nutrition, Article ID 126929, 6 pages, (2013) doi:10.5402/2013/126929
351. G Kolata. How important is dietary calcium in preventing osteoporosis? Science; 1986: 233 (4763), 519-520. [DOI:10.1126/science.3726543], References Full Text (PDF)
352. Lousuebsakul-Matthews, Vichuda; Thorpe, Donna L.; Knutsen, Raymond; et al. Legumes and meat analogues consumption are associated with hip fracture risk independently of meat intake among Caucasian men and women: the Adventist Health Study-2; Public Health Nutrition;2014; 17, 10, 2333-2343
353. Deborah E Sellmeyer, Katie L Stone, Anthony Sebastian, Steven R Cummings. A high ratio of dietary animal to vegetable protein increases the rate of bone loss and the risk of fracture in postmenopausal women; Am J Clin Nutr ; 2001; 73 ,1, 118-122
354. Kubena, Karen S et al. Nutrition and the Immune System; Journal of the American Dietetic Association; 1996; 96 , 11 , 1156 - 1164 DOI: http://dx.doi.org/10.1016/S0002-8223(96)00297-0
355. Report from the Infant Feeding Information Team, Blackpool and North Lancashire: (February 2012)
356. Wonders of breast milk: www.007b.com/wonders_breastmilk.php
357. Web MD, Breastfeeding vs. Formula Feeding: http://www.webmd.com/baby/breastfeeding-vs-formula-feeding
358. Christakis DA. Breastfeeding and Cognition: Can IQ Tip the Scale?. JAMA Pediatr;2013;167(9):796-797. doi:10.1001/jamapediatrics.2013.470.
359. Belfort MB, Rifas-Shiman SL, Kleinman KP, et al. Infant Feeding and Childhood Cognition at Ages 3 and 7 Years: Effects of Breastfeeding Duration and Exclusivity. JAMA Pediatr. 2013;167(9):836-844. doi:10.1001/jamapediatrics.2013.455.
360. Jain A, Concato J, Leventhal JM. How good is the evidence linking breastfeeding and intelligence? Pediatrics; 2002;109(6): 1044-1053. Link to Article

References

361. Anderson JW, Johnstone BM, Remley DT. Breast-feeding and cognitive development: a meta-analysis. Am J Clin Nutr; 1999;70(4): 525-535.
362. Drane DL, Logemann JA. A critical evaluation of the evidence on the association between type of infant feeding and cognitive development. Paediatr Perinat Epidemiol; 2000;14(4):349-356.
363. Warensjo E, Jansson JH, Berglund L, et al. Estimated intake of milk fat is negatively associated with cardiovascular risk factors and does not increase the risk of a first acute myocardial infarction. Br J Nutr; 2004;91:635–642.
364. M Kestin, I L Rouse, R A Correll, and P J Nestel. Cardiovascular disease risk factors in free-living men: comparison of two prudent diets, one based on lactoovovegetarianism and the other allowing lean meat. Am J Clin Nutr; 1989; 50, 2. 280-287
365. Sacks FM, Ornish D, Rosner B, McLanahan S, Castelli WP, Kass EH. Plasma Lipoprotein Levels in Vegetarians: The Effect of Ingestion of Fats From Dairy Products. JAMA; 1985;254(10):1337-1341. doi: 10.1001/jama.1985.03360100087019.
366. World Heart Federation: www.world-heart-federation.org/cardiovascular-health/cardiovascular-disease-risk-factors/diet/
367. American Academy of Pediatrics, Commitee on nutrition. The Use of Whole Cow's Milk in Infancy. Pediatrics; 1992; 89, 6. pp. 1105 -1109.
368. American Academy of Pediatrics, Commitee on Nutrition. Iron fortified formulas. Pediatrics; 1971;45-55
369. Jonathon L. Maguire, Gerald Lebovic, Sharmilaa Kandasamy, Marina Khovratovich, Muhammad Mamdani, Catherine S. Birken, Patricia C. Parkin. The Relationship Between Cow's Milk and Stores of Vitamin D and Iron in Early Childhood; Pediatrics; 2013; 131:1 e144-e151; doi: 10.1542/peds.2012-1793
370. National Survey of Family Growth, www.cdc.gov/nchs/data/factsheets/factsheet_nsfg.pdf
371. J.E. Chavarro, et al. "A Prospective Study of Dairy Foods Intake and Anovulatory Infertility." Human Reproduction; 2007; 22, 5, 1340-1347.
372. Lanou AJ, Berkow SE, Barnard ND. Calcium, dairy products, and bone health in children and young adults: a reevaluation of the evidence. Pediatrics; 2005;115:736–743.
373. Cramer DW, Harlow BL, Willett WC, Welch WR, Bell DA, Scully RE, Ng WG, Knapp RC. Galactose consumption and metabolism in relation to the risk of ovarian cancer. Lancet; 1989;2(8654):66-71.

References

374. Ganmaa D, Sato A. The possible role of female sex hormones in milk from pregnant cows in the development of breast, ovarian, and corpus uteri cancers. Med Hypotheses; 2005; 65:1028–37.
375. World Cancer Research Fund, American Institute for Cancer Research. Food, nutrition, physical activity, and the prevention of cancer: a global perspective. Washington DC: AICR, (2007).
376. Giovannucci E, Rimm EB, Wolk A, et al. Calcium and fructose intake in relation to risk of prostate cancer. Cancer Res; 1998; 58:442–447.
377. Giovannucci E, Liu Y, Platz EA, Stampfer MJ, Willett WC. Risk factors for prostate cancer incidence and progression in the Health Professionals Follow-up Study. International Journal of Cancer; 2007; 121:1571–78.
378. Dunaif GE, Campbell TC. Relative contribution of dietary protein level and aflatoxin B1 dose in generation of presumptive preneoplastic foci in rat liver. J Natl Cancer Inst;1987;78(2):365-9.
379. Ben Spencer. 135 diabetes amputations every week: Obesity blamed for 17% rise in operations. The Daily Mail. (July 2015)
380. Saukkonen T, Virtanen SM, Karppinen M, et al. Significance of cow's milk protein antibodies as risk factor for childhood IDDM: interaction with dietary cow's milk intake and HLA-DQB1 genotype. Childhood Diabetes in Finland Study Group. Dibetologia; 1998;41:72–78.
381. Kimpimaki T, Erkkola M, Korhonen S, et al. Short-term exclusive breastfeeding predisposes young children with increased genetic risk of type I diabetes to progressive beta-cell autoimmunity. Diabetologia;. 2001;44:63–69.
382. Eidelman AI, Schanler RJ. Policy statement: breastfeeding and the use of human milk. From the American Academy of Pediatrics. Pediatrics; 2012;129:827–841.
383. Lamb MM, Miller M, Seifert JA, Frederiksen B, Kroehl M, Rewers M, Norris JM. ; The effect of childhood cow's milk intake and HLA-DR genotype on risk of islet autoimmunity and type 1 diabetes: The Diabetes Autoimmunity Study in the Young. Pediatr Diabetes; 2014; doi: 10.1111/pedi.12115.
384. Honeyman MC, Stone NL & Harrison LC. T-cell epitopes in type 1 diabetes autoantigen tyrosine phosphatase IA-2: potential for mimicry with rotavirus and other environmental agents. Molecular Medicine; 1998; 4 231–239.
385. Knip M, Veijola R, Virtanen SM, Hyoty H, Vaarala O & Akerblom HK. Environmental triggers and determinants of type 1 diabetes. Diabetes; 2005; 54 (Suppl 2) S125–S136. (doi:10.2337/diabetes.54.suppl_2.S125).

References

386. Johnston CS & Monte WC. Infant formula ingestion is associated with the development of diabetes in the BB/Wor rat. Life Sciences; 2000; 66 1501–1507. (doi:10.1016/S0024-3205(00)00467-7).
387. Honeyman MC, Stone NL & Harrison LC. T-cell epitopes in type 1 diabetes autoantigen tyrosine phosphatase IA-2: potential for mimicry with rotavirus and other environmental agents. Molecular Medicine; 1998; 4 231–239.
388. Chen Y1, Jiang YX, Yi L, Miu AZ, Zhang SJ, Wu JH, Zhang SH. Excessive milk intake as a risk factor, probably associated with oxidative stress, in experimental naphthalene-initiated cataract in rats; Ophthalmic Res; 2012;47(2):87-97. doi: 10.1159/000330504.
389. Obara Y. The oxidative stress in the cataract formation]. Nihon Ganka Gakkai Zasshi; 1995; 99(12):1303-41.
390. Birlouez-Aragon I, Ravelontseheno L, Villate-Cathelineau B, Cathelineau G, Abitbol G. ; Disturbed galactose metabolism in elderly and diabetic humans is associated with cataract formation. J Nutr. 1993;123(8):1370-6
391. Szeto YT, Kwok TC, Benzie IF. Effects of a long-term vegetarian diet on biomarkers of antioxidants status and cardiovascular disease risk. Nutrition; 2004;20:863–866.
392. Ornish D, Brown SE, Scherwitz LW, et al. Can lifestyle changes reverse coronary heart disease? Lancet; 1990;336:129–133.
393. Bernstein, Bradley E.; Meissner, Alexander; Lander,Eric S. The Mammalian Epigenome. Cell; 2007; 128 (4): 669–681. doi:10.1016/j.cell.2007.01.033. PMID 17320505.
394. Eva Bianconi, Allison Piovesan, Federica Facchin, Alina Beraudi, Raffaella Casadei, Flavia Frabetti, Lorenza Vitale, Maria Chiara Pelleri, Simone Tassani, Francesco Piva, Soledad Perez-Amodio, Pierluigi Strippoli, and Silvia Canaider. An estimation of the number of cells in the human body; Annals of Human Biology; 2013; Vol. 40, No. 6 , Pages 463-471 (doi:10.3109/03014460.2013.807878)
395. Pereira, S. L.; Rodrigues, A. S.; Sousa, M. I.; Correia, M.; Perestrelo, T.; Ramalho-Santos, J."From gametogenesis and stem cells to cancer: common metabolic themes. Human Reproduction Update; 2014; 20 (6): 924–943. doi:10.1093/humupd/dmu034. ISSN 1355-4786.
396. Watson, J. D., & Crick, F. H. C. A structure for deoxyribose nucleic acid. Nature; 1953; 171, 737–738
397. Crick, F. "Central dogma of molecular biology.". Nature; 1970; 227 (5258): 561–3. Bibcode:1970Natur.227..561C. doi:10.1038/227561a0. PMID 4913914.

References

398. Philip Ball. DNA: Celebrate the unknowns; Nature; 2013; 496, 419–420 doi:10.1038/496419a
399. Wikipedia.org Stem cells en.wikipedia.org/wiki/Stem_cell
400. Berg JM, Tymoczko JL, Stryer L. Biochemistry. 5th edition. New York: W H Freeman; (2002). Section 2.4, Cells Can Respond to Changes in Their Environments. Available from: http://www.ncbi.nlm.nih.gov/books/NBK22568/
401. Bygren LO, Edvinsson S, Broström G: Change in food availability during pregnancy: is it related to adult sudden death from cerebro- and cardiovascular disease in offspring. Am J Hum Biol; 2000; 12: 447–453.
402. Waterland RA, Jirtle RL. "Transposable elements: targets for early nutritional effects on epigenetic gene regulation", Mol Cell Biol; 2003; 23: 5293–5300. PMID 12861015
403. Kaufman, Peter B.; Duke, James A.; Brielmann, Harry; Boik, John; Hoyt, James E. A Comparative Survey of Leguminous Plants as Sources of the Isoflavones, Genistein and Daidzein: Implications for Human Nutrition and Health. The Journal of Alternative and Complementary Medicine; 1997; 3,1, 7–12. doi:10.1089/acm.1997.3.7. PMID 9395689.
404. Scanlan RA. Formation and occurrence of nitrosamines in food. Cancer Res; 1983;43,5 ,2435s-2440s.
405. Dolinoy DC, Weidman JR, Waterland RA, Jirtle RL. "Maternal genistein alters coat color and protects Avy mouse offspring from obesity by modifying the fetal epigenome", Environ Health Perspect; 2006;114: 567–572. PMID 16581547
406. Dolinoy DC, Huang D, Jirtle RL. "Maternal nutrient supplementation counteracts bisphenol A-induced DNA hypomethylation in early development", PNAS 104: 13056–13061. (2007) PMID 17670942
407. American Society of Human Genetics. "Humans, chimpanzees and monkeys share DNA but not gene regulatory mechanisms." ScienceDaily. Sciencedaily, 6 November 2012. <www.sciencedaily.com/releases/2012/11/121106201124.htm>
408. Zhou X, Cain CE, Myrthil M, Lewellen N, Michelini K, Davenport ER, Stephens M, Pritchard JK, and Gilad Y. Epigenetic Modifications are Associated with Inter-species Gene Expression Variation in Primates. Genome Biology;. 2014; 15:547.
409. Varga, Andrew W; Kishi, Akifumi; Mantua, Janna; Lim, Jason; Koushyk, Viachaslau; Leibert, David P; Osorio, Ricardo S; Rapoport, David M; Ayappa,. Apnea-induced rapid eye movement sleep disruption impairs human spatial navigational memory; Journal of neuroscience; 2014; 34(44):14571-14577.

References

410. E. Juulia Paavonen, Katri Räikkönen, Jari Lahti, Niina Komsi, Kati Heinonen, Anu-Katriina Pesonen, Anna-Liisa Järvenpää, Timo Strandberg, Eero Kajantie, Tarja Porkka-Heiskanen. Short Sleep Duration and Behavioral Symptoms of Attention-Deficit/Hyperactivity Disorder in Healthy 7- to 8-Year-Old Children; Pediatrics; 2009; 123,5, e857-e864 (doi: 10.1542/peds.2008-2164)
411. Patel SR, Ayas NT, Malhotra MR, White DP, Schernhammer ES, Speizer FE, Stampfer MJ, Hu FB. A prospective study of sleep duration and mortality risk in women. Sleep; 2004;27,3,440-4.
412. Sigurdson K, Ayas N. The public health and safety consequences of sleep disorders. Canadian J Physiol Pharmacol; 2007; 85,179-183.
413. Hublin C, Partinen M, Koskenvuo M, Kaprio J. Sleep and mortality: a population-based 22-year follow-up study. Sleep; 2007;30,10,1245-53.
414. O'Connor, George T; Caffo, Brian; Newman, Anne B; Quan, Stuart F; Rapoport, David M; Redline, Susan; Resnick, Helaine E; Samet, Jonathan; Shahar, Eyal. Prospective Study of Sleep-Disordered Breathing and Hypertension: The Sleep Heart Health Study. American journal of respiratory & critical care medicine; 2009;179(12):1159-1164.
415. Matthews KA, Zheng H, Kravitz HM, et al. Are Inflammatory and Coagulation Biomarkers Related to Sleep Characteristics in Mid-Life Women?: Study of Women's Health Across the Nation Sleep Study. Sleep. 2010;33(12):1649-1655
416. Morris AA, Zhao L, Ahmed Y, Stoyanova N, De Staercke C, Hooper WC, Gibbons G, Din-Dzietham R, Quyyumi A, Vaccarino V. Association between depression and inflammation--differences by race and sex: the META-Health study. Psychosom Med; 2011;73,6:462-8. doi: 10.1097/PSY.0b013e318222379c
417. Ajani UA, Ford ES, McGuire LC. Distribution of lifestyle and emerging risk factors by 10-year risk for coronary heart disease. Eur J Cardiovasc Prev Rehabil; 2006;13(5):745-52
418. Centers for Disease Control And Prevention: www.cdc.gov/search.do?subset=&queryText=c+reactive+protein+heart+disease
419. Poor Sleep Quality Increases Inflammation, Community Study Finds: shared.web.emory.edu/whsc/news/releases/2010/11/poor-sleep-quality-increases-inflammation-study-finds.html
420. Taheri S, Lin L, Austin D, Young T, Mignot E. Short sleep duration is associated with reduced leptin, elevated ghrelin, and increased body mass index. PLoS Med; 2004; 1:e62.
421. Spiegel K, Tasali E, Penev P, Van Cauter E. Brief communication: Sleep curtailment in healthy young men is associated with decreased leptin

References

levels, elevated ghrelin levels, and increased hunger and appetite. Ann Intern Med; 2004; 141:846-50.
422. Taheri S. The link between short sleep duration and obesity: we should recommend more sleep to prevent obesity. Arch Dis Child; 2006; 91:881-4.
423. Nedeltcheva AV, Kilkus JM, Imperial J, Kasza K, Schoeller DA, Penev PD. Sleep curtailment is accompanied by increased intake of calories from snacks. Am J Clin Nutr; 2009; 89:126-33.
424. Imaki M, Hatanaka Y, Ogawa Y, Yoshida Y, Tanada S. An epidemiological study on relationship between the hours of sleep and life style factors in Japanese factory workers. J Physiol Anthropol Appl Human Sci; 2002; 21:115-20
425. Patel SR, Malhotra A, White DP, Gottlieb DJ, Hu FB. Association between reduced sleep and weight gain in women. Am J Epidemiol; 2006; 164:947-54.
426. Zizi F, Jean-Louis G, Brown CD, Ogedegbe G, Boutin-Foster C, McFarlane SI. Sleep Duration and the Risk of Diabetes Mellitus: Epidemiologic Evidence and Pathophysiologic Insights. Current diabetes reports; 2010;10(1):43-47. doi:10.1007/s11892-009-0082-x.
427. Broussard JL, Ehrmann DA, Van Cauter E, Tasali E, Brady MJ. Impaired insulin signaling in human adipocytes after experimental sleep restriction: a randomized, crossover study. Ann Intern Med; 2012 Oct 16;157(8):549-57.doi:10.7326/0003-4819-157-8-201210160-00005.
428. Mah CD, Mah KE, Kezirian EJ, Dement WC. The Effects of Sleep Extension on the Athletic Performance of Collegiate Basketball Players. Sleep; 2011;34(7):943-950. doi:10.5665/SLEEP.1132.
429. Reilly T, Piercy M. The effect of partial sleep deprivation on weight-lifting performance. Ergonomics; 1994;37:107–15.
430. Edwards BJ, Waterhouse J. Effects of one night of partial sleep deprivation upon diurnal rhythms of accuracy and consistency in throwing darts. Chronobiol Int;2009;26:756–68.
431. Kline CE, Durstine JL, Davis JM, et al. Circadian variation in swim performance. J Appl Physiol;. 2007;102:641–9.
429. Cappuccio FP; D'Elia L; Strazzullo P; Miller MA. Sleep duration and all-cause mortality: a systematic review and meta-analysis of prospective studies. SLEEP 2010; 33,5, 585-592.
430. Kingman P. Strohl, Daniel B. Brown, Nancy Collop, Charles George, Ronald Grunstein, Fang Han, Lawrence Kline, Atul Malhotra, Alan Pack, Barbara Phillips, Daniel Rodenstein, Richard Schwab, Terri Weaver, and Kevin Wilson; on behalf of the ATS Ad Hoc Committee on

References

Sleep Apnea, Sleepiness, and Driving Risk in Noncommercial Drivers. An Official American Thoracic Society Clinical Practice Guideline: Sleep Apnea, Sleepiness, and Driving Risk in Noncommercial Drivers. An Update of a 1994 Statement. American Thoracic Society Documents, (2012).

431. US Department of Transportation, National Highway Traffic Safety Administration, National Center on Sleep Disorders Research, National Heart Lung and Blood Institute. Drowsy driving and automobile crashes [National Highway Traffic Safety Administration Web Site]. Accessed November 24, 2014.

432. Kamdar BB, Kaplan KA, Kezirian EJ, Dement WC. The impact of extended sleep on daytime alertness, vigilance, and mood. Sleep Med; 2004;5:441–8.

433. Belenky G, Wesensten N, Thorne D, et al. Patterns of performance degradation and restoration during sleep restriction and subsequent recovery: a sleep dose-response study. J Sleep Res; 2003;12:1–12

434. 761

435. Kathelijne Koops,*, William C. McGrew, Tetsuro Matsuzawa andLeslie A. Knapp. Terrestrial nest-building by wild chimpanzees (Pan troglodytes): Implications for the tree-to-ground sleep transition in early hominins; American Journal of Physical Anthropology; 2012; 148,3, pages 351–361

436. Institute of Medicine. Sleep Disorders and Sleep Deprivation: An Unmet Public Health Problem. Washington, DC: The National Academies Press; (2006).

437. A. Roger Ekirch. At Day's Close: Night in Times Past; Norton (2005)

438. Wehr, T. A. "In short photoperiods, human sleep is biphasic". Journal of Sleep Research 1; 1992; (2): 103–107. doi:10.1111/j.1365-2869.1992.tb00019.x. PMID 10607034.

439. Russell Foster: Why do we sleep? www.ted.com/talks/russell_foster_why_do_we_sleep?language=en

440. Gillberg M, Kecklund G, Axelsson J, Akerstedt T. The effects of a short daytime nap after restricted night sleep; Sleep; 1996;19(7):570-5

441. Strategies for Getting Enough Sleep - NHLBI, NIH: www.nhlbi.nih.gov/health/health-topics/topics/sdd/strategies

442. neuroplasticity | biology | Encyclopedia Britannica www.britannica.com/EBchecked/topic/410552/neuroplasticity

443. Dawkins, R. The Ancestor's Tale: A Pilgrimage to the Dawn of Evolution, Houghton Mifflin Harcourt, (2005) ISBN 978-0-618-61916-0

References

444. Timeline of human evolution: en.m.wikipedia.org/wiki/Timeline_of_human_evolution
445. Sporns, O. Networks of the Brain. MIT Press. p. 143. (2010) ISBN 978-0-262-01469-4.
446. Başar, E. Brain-Body-Mind in the Nebulous Cartesian System: A Holistic Approach by Oscillations. Springer. p. 225. (2010) ISBN 978-1-4419-6134-1.
447. Shepherd, GM. Neurobiology. Oxford University Press. p. 3. (1994) ISBN 978-0-19-508843-4.
448. Lui, J. H.; Hansen, D. V.; Kriegstein, A. R. "Development and Evolution of the Human Neocortex". Cell; 2011; 146,1, 18–36. doi:10.1016/j.cell.2011.06.030. PMC 3610574. PMID 21729779
449. Wikipedia-Fear: en.wikipedia.org/wiki/Fear
450. Goldstein A, Lowery PJ. "Effect of the opiate antagonist naloxone on body temperature in rats". Life Sciences; 1975; 17 (6): 927–31. doi: 10.1016/0024-3205(75)90445-2. PMID 1195988.
451. Cotman CW, Berchtold NC. "Exercise: a behavioral intervention to enhance brain health and plasticity". Trends Neurosci;2002; 25 (6): 295–301. doi:10.1016/S0166-2236(02)02143-4. PMID 12086747.
452. Zigova T, Pencea V, Wiegand SJ, Luskin MB. "Intraventricular administration of BDNF increases the number of newly generated neurons in the adult olfactory bulb". Mol. Cell. Neurosci; 1998; 11 (4): 234–45. doi:10.1006/mcne.1998.0684. PMID 9675054.
453. Benraiss A, Chmielnicki E, Lerner K, Roh D, Goldman SA. "Adenoviral brain-derived neurotrophic factor induces both neostriatal and olfactory neuronal recruitment from endogenous progenitor cells in the adult forebrain". J. Neurosci; 2001; 21 (17): 6718–31. PMID 11517261.
454. Pencea V, Bingaman KD, Wiegand SJ, Luskin MB. "Infusion of brain-derived neurotrophic factor into the lateral ventricle of the adult rat leads to new neurons in the parenchyma of the striatum, septum, thalamus, and hypothalamus". J. Neurosci; 2001; 21 (17): 6706–17. PMID 11517260.
455. Acheson A, Conover JC, Fandl JP, DeChiara TM, Russell M, Thadani A et al. "A BDNF autocrine loop in adult sensory neurons prevents cell death". Nature; 1995; 374 (6521): 450–3. doi:10.1038/374450a0. PMID 7700353.
456. Huang EJ, Reichardt LF. "Neurotrophins: Roles in Neuronal Development and Function". Annu. Rev. Neurosci; 2001; 24: 677–736. doi:10.1146/annurev.neuro.24.1.677. PMC 2758233. PMID 11520916.

References

457. Bekinschtein P, Cammarota M, Katche C, Slipczuk L, Rossato JI, Goldin A et al. "BDNF is essential to promote persistence of long-term memory storage". Proc. Natl. Acad. Sci. U.S.A.; 2008; 105 (7): 2711–6. doi:10.1073/pnas.0711863105. PMC 2268201. PMID 18263738.
458. Yamada K, Nabeshima T. "Brain-derived neurotrophic factor/TrkB signaling in memory processes". J. Pharmacol. Sci; 2003; 91 (4): 267–70. doi:10.1254/jphs.91.267. PMID 12719654.
459. Lee IM, Shiroma EJ, Lobelo F, et al. Effect of physical inactivity on major non-communicable diseases worldwide: an analysis of burden of disease and life expectancy. Lancet; 2012; 380:219.
460. Owen N, Sparling PB, Healy GN, et al. Sedentary behavior: emerging evidence for a new health risk. Mayo Clin Proc; 2010; 85:1138.
461. Herring MP, O'Connor PJ, Dishman RK. The effect of exercise training on anxiety symptoms among patients: a systematic review. Arch Intern Med; 2010; 170:321.
462. Peterson DM. Overview of the benefits and risks of exercise. Accessed Feb 1, 2015.
463. Lawton BA, Rose SB, Raina Elley C, et al. Exercise on prescription for women aged 40-74 recruited through primary care: two year randomised controlled trial. Br J Sports Med; 2009; 43:120
464. Kodama S, Saito K, Tanaka S, et al. Cardiorespiratory fitness as a quantitative predictor of all-cause mortality and cardiovascular events in healthy men and women: a meta-analysis. JAMA; 2009; 301:2024.
465. Slentz CA, Duscha BD, Johnson JL, et al. Effects of the amount of exercise on body weight, body composition, and measures of central obesity: STRRIDE--a randomized controlled study. Arch Intern Med; 2004; 164:31.
466. Irwin ML, Yasui Y, Ulrich CM, et al. Effect of exercise on total and intra-abdominal body fat in postmenopausal women: a randomized controlled trial. JAMA; 2003; 289:323.
467. Leitzmann MF, Park Y, Blair A, et al. Physical activity recommendations and decreased risk of mortality. Arch Intern Med; 2007; 167:2453.
468. The benefits of physical activity. Centers for Disease Control and Prevention. Accessed February 1, 2015. www.cdc.gov/physicalactivity/everyone/health/index.html
469. Wannamethee SG, Shaper AG, Alberti KG. Physical activity, metabolic factors, and the incidence of coronary heart disease and type 2 diabetes. Arch Intern Med; 2000; 160:2108.

References

470. Irwin ML, Yasui Y, Ulrich CM, et al. Effect of exercise on total and intra-abdominal body fat in postmenopausal women: a randomized controlled trial. JAMA; 2003; 289:323.
471. Smith, JK; Dykes, R; Douglas, JE; Krishnaswamy, G; Berk, S. "Long-term exercise and atherogenic activity of blood mononuclear cells in persons at risk of developing ischemic heart disease.". JAMA: the Journal of the American Medical Association; 1999; 281 (18): 1722–7. doi:10.1001/jama.281.18.1722. PMID 10328073.
472. McFarlin, BK; Flynn, MG; Phillips, MD; Stewart, LK; Timmerman, KL. "Chronic resistance exercise training improves natural killer cell activity in older women.". The journals of gerontology. Series A, Biological sciences and medical sciences; 2005; 60 (10): 1315–8. doi:10.1093/gerona/60.10.1315. PMID 16282566.
473. Stewart, LK; Flynn, MG; Campbell, WW; Craig, BA; Robinson, JP; McFarlin, BK; Timmerman, KL; Coen, PM; Felker, J; Talbert, E. "Influence of exercise training and age on CD14+ cell-surface expression of toll-like receptor 2 and 4.". Brain, behavior, and immunity ; 2005;19 (5): 389–97. doi:10.1016/j.bbi.2005.04.003. PMID 15963685.
474. Lovejoy CO, Johanson DC, Coppens Y. Hominid lower limbbones recovered from Hadar formation. Am J Phys Anthr; 1982; 38:757-780
475. Leaky MD, Hay RL. Pliocene footprints in the Laetolil Beds at laetoli, northern Tanzania. Nature; 1979; 278:317-323
476. Krantz GS, Brain size and hunting ability in earliest man. Current Anthropology; 1968; 9:450-451.
477. Watanabe H. Running, creeping and climbing: A new ecological and evolutionary perspective on human locomotion. Mankind; 1971; 8:1-13.
478. Schapera I. The Khoisan peoples of South Africa: Bushman and Hottentots. London: Routledge and Kegan Paul. (1930)
479. Bennett WC, Zingg RM. The TArahumara: An Indian tribe of Northern Mexico. Chicago: University of Chicago Press. (1935)
480. Lowie RH. Notes on Shoshonean ethnography. Anthropological papers of the American Museum Of Natural History; 1924; 20 pt 3.
481. Sollas WJ. Ancient hunters and their modern representatives. New York: Macmillan. (1924)
482. Eichna LW, Park CR, Nelson N, Horvath SM, Palmes, ED. Thermal regulation during acclimitisation to a hot, dry environment. Am J Phys; 1950; 163:585-587.
483. Lovejoy CO. Evolution of human walking. Sci Am; 1988; 259:118-125
484. Rodman PS, McHenry HM, MAloiy GO. Energetics and the origin of hominid bipedalism. Am J Phys Anthrop; 1980; 52:103-106.

References

485. Tucker VA. The cost of moving about. Am Sci; 1975; 63:413-419
486. Arbitoi MM: Effect of posture and locomotion on energy expenditure. Am J Phys Anthrop; 1988; 77:191-199
487. David R. Carrier, A. K. Kapoor, Tasuku Kimura, Martin K. Nickels, Satwanti, Eugenie C. Scott, Joseph K. So and Erik Trinkaus. The Energetic Paradox of Human Running and Hominid Evolution [and Comments and Reply]; Current Anthropology; 1984; 25, 4, 483-495
488. Krantz GS, Brain size and hunting ability in earliest man. Current Anthropology; 1968; 9:450-451.
489. Bramble DM, Carrier DR. Running and breathing in mammals. Science; 1983; 219:251-256
490. Eichna LW, Park CR, Nelson N, Horvath SM, Palmes, ED. Thermal regulation during acclimitisation to a hot, dry environment. Am J Phys; 1950, 163:585 587.
491. Schmidt-Nielsen K. Desert animals: Physiological problems of heat and water. New York: Oxford University Press. (1964)
492. Wheeler PE. The influence of bipedalism on the energy and water budgets of early hominids. J Hum Evol; 1991; 21:117-136.
493. Wheeler PE. The influence of the loss of functional body hair on the water budgets of early hominids. J Hum Evol; 1992; 23:379-388
494. Foley R, Lee PC. Finite social space, evolutionary pathways and reconstructing hominid behaviour. Science; 1989; 243:901-906.
495. Horton ES. Exercise and physical training: Effects on insulin sensitivity and glucose metabolism. Diabetes Metab Rev; 1986; 2:1-17.
496. Fluckey JD, Hickey MS, Brambrink JK, Hart KK, Alexander K, Craig BW. Effects of resistance exercise on glucose control in normal and glucose intolerant subjects. J Appl Phys; 1994; 77:1087-1092.
497. Kriska AM, Blair SN, Pereira MA: The potential role of physical activity in the prevention of non insulin dependant diabetes mellitus: The epidemiological evidence. Exerc Sports Sci Rev; 1994; 22: 121-143.
498. Bergstrom J, Hemansen L, Hultman E, Saltin B. Diet, muscle glycogen, and physical performance. Acta Physiologica Scandinavica; 1967; 71:140-150.
499. Karlsson J, Saltin B. Diet, muscle glycogen, and endurance performance. J Appl Phys; 1971; 31:203-206
500. Gollnick PD, Piehl K, Saubert CW, Armstrong RB, Saltin B. Diet, exercise and glycogen changesin human muscle fibers. J Appl Phys; 1972; 33:421-425
501. David R. Carrier, A. K. Kapoor, Tasuku Kimura, Martin K. Nickels, Satwanti, Eugenie C. Scott, Joseph K. So and Erik Trinkaus. The

References

Energetic Paradox of Human Running and Hominid Evolution [and Comments and Reply]; Current Anthropology; 1984; 25, 4, 483-495

502. Huang EJ, Reichardt LF. "Neurotrophins: Roles in Neuronal Development and Function". Annu. Rev. Neurosci; 2001;24, 677–736. doi:10.1146/annurev.neuro.24.1.677. PMC 2758233. PMID 11520916.

503. Acheson A, Conover JC, Fandl JP, DeChiara TM, Russell M, Thadani A et al. A BDNF autocrine loop in adult sensory neurons prevents cell death. Nature; 1995; 374,6521, 450–3. doi:10.1038/374450a0. PMID 7700353.

504. Pérez-Escamilla, Rafael et al. Dietary Energy Density and Body Weight in Adults and Children: A Systematic Review; Journal of the Academy of Nutrition and Dietetics; 2012; 112 , 5 , 671 - 684

505. Rolls BJ, Drewnowski A, Ledikwe JH. Changing the energy density of the diet as a strategy for weight management; J Am Diet Assoc; 2005; 105(5 Suppl 1):S98-103.

506. Drewnowski A. The role of energy density; Lipids; 2003; 38(2):109-15.

507. American Institute for Cancer Research (AICR); Food, Nutrition, Physical Activity, and the Prevention of Cancer: a Global Perspective

508. Scanlan RA. Formation and occurrence of nitrosamines in food. Cancer Res; 1983;43,5 ,2435s-2440s.

509. Strang, J., Drummond, C., McNeill, A. et al. Addictions, dependence and substance misuse In: Davies, S Annual Report of the Chief Medical Officer 2013: Public Mental Health priorities: investing in the evidence. (2014)

510. The Effects Of Alcohol On The Liver: https://www.drinkaware.co.uk/check-the-facts/health-effects-of-alcohol/effects-on-the-body/alcohol-and-your-liver

511. Tordoff MG, Alleva AM. Oral stimulation with aspartame increases hunger. Physiol Behav. 1990;47,3:555-9.

512. Brown RJ, de Banate MA, Rother KI. Artificial sweeteners: a systematic review of metabolic effects in youth. Int J Pediatr Obes. 2010;5,4:305-12. doi: 10.3109/17477160903497027.

513. Slutsker L, Hoesly FC, Miller L, Williams LP, Watson JC, Fleming DW. "Eosinophilia-myalgia syndrome associated with exposure to tryptophan from a single manufacturer". 1990;JAMA 264,2: 213–7. doi: 10.1001/jama.264.2.213. PMID 2355442.

514. Hung HC, Joshipura KJ, Jiang R, et al. Fruit and vegetable intake and risk of major chronic disease. J Natl Cancer Inst; 2004; 96:1577–84.

515. He FJ, Nowson CA, Lucas M, MacGregor GA. Increased consumption of fruit and vegetables is related to a reduced risk of coronary heart

disease: meta-analysis of cohort studies. J Hum Hypertens; 2007; 21:717–28.
516. He FJ, Nowson CA, MacGregor GA. Fruit and vegetable consumption and stroke: meta-analysis of cohort studies. Lancet; 2006; 367:320–26.
517. Appel LJ, Moore TJ, Obarzanek E, et al. A clinical trial of the effects of dietary patterns on blood pressure. DASH Collaborative Research Group. N Engl J Med; 1997; 336:1117–24.
518. World Cancer Research Fund, American Institute for Cancer Research. Food, Nutrition, Physical Activity, and the Prevention of Cancer: a Global Perspective. Washington DC: AICR, (2007)
519. Giovannucci E, Liu Y, Platz EA, Stampfer MJ, Willett WC. Risk factors for prostate cancer incidence and progression in the Health Professionals Follow-up Study. Int J Cancer; 2007; 121:1571–78.
520. Kavanaugh CJ, Trumbo PR, Ellwood KC. The U.S. Food and Drug Administration's evidence-based review for qualified health claims: tomatoes, lycopene, and cancer. J Natl Cancer Inst; 2007; 99:1074–85
521. Christen WG, Liu S, Schaumberg DA, Buring JE. Fruit and vegetable intake and the risk of cataract in women. Am J Clin Nutr; 2005; 81:1417–22.
522. Moeller SM, Taylor A, Tucker KL, et al. Overall adherence to the dietary guidelines for Americans is associated with reduced prevalence of early age-related nuclear lens opacities in women. J Nutr; 2004; 134:1812–19.
523. Cho E, Seddon JM, Rosner B, Willett WC, Hankinson SE. Prospective study of intake of fruits, vegetables, vitamins, and carotenoids and risk of age-related maculopathy. Arch Ophthalmol; 2004; 122:883–92.
524. Christen WG, Liu S, Glynn RJ, Gaziano JM, Buring JE. Dietary carotenoids, vitamins C and E, and risk of cataract in women: A prospective study. Arch Ophthalmol; 2008; 126:102–109.
525. U.S. Department of Agriculture and U.S. Department of Health and Human Services. Dietary Guidelines for Americans, 2010. 7th Edition, Washington, DC: U.S. Government Printing Office, (2010).
526. Vartanian LR, Schwartz MB, Brownell KD. Effects of Soft Drink Consumption on Nutrition and Health: A Systematic Review and Meta-Analysis. American Journal of Public Health; 2007;97,4,667-675. doi: 10.2105/AJPH.2005.083782.
527. Lembo A, Camilleri M. Chronic constipation. N Engl J Med; 2003; 349:1360–68.
528. American Institute for Cancer Research (AICR); Food, Nutrition, Physical Activity, and the Prevention of Cancer: a Global Perspective

References

529. Aldoori WH, Giovannucci EL, Rockett HR, Sampson L, Rimm EB, Willett WC. A prospective study of dietary fiber types and symptomatic diverticular disease in men. J Nutr; 1998; 128:714–19.
530. American Institute for Cancer Research (AICR); Food, Nutrition, Physical Activity, and the Prevention of Cancer: a Global Perspective
531. Kerstetter JE, O'Brien KO, Insogna KL. Low protein intake: the impact on calcium and bone homeostasis in humans. J Nutr; 2003;133:855S-61S.
532. Physicians committee for responsible medicine: www.pcrm.org/health/diets/vsk/vegetarian-starter-kit-calcium
533. Weaver CM, Plawecki KL. Dietary calcium: adequacy of a vegetarian diet. Am J Clin Nutr; 1994;59 (suppl):1238S-1241S.
534. Weaver CM, Heaney RP, Nickel KP, et al. Calcium bioavailability from high oxalate vegetables: Chinese vegetables, sweet potatoes, and rhubarb. J Food Sci; 1997;62:524-525.
535. Jump DB, Clarke SD. Regulation of gene expression by dietary fat. Annu Rev Nutr; 1999;19, 63–90.
536. Waterland RA, Jirtle RL. "Transposable elements: targets for early nutritional effects on epigenetic gene regulation", Mol Cell Biol; 2003; 23: 5293–5300. PMID 12861015
537. Duca FA, Swartz TD, Sakar Y, Covasa M Increased Oral Detection, but Decreased Intestinal Signaling for Fats in Mice Lacking Gut Microbiota. PLOS ONE (2012) 7(6): e39748.
538. Sarr, M.G., Billington, C.J., Brancatisano, R. et al. The EMPOWER Study: Randomized, Prospective, Double-Blind, Multicenter Trial of Vagal Blockade to Induce Weight Loss in Morbid Obesity. OBES SURG (2012) 22: 1771.
539. Paul E. Sawchenko, Richard M. Gold, Sarah Fryer Leibowitz, Evidence for vagal involvement in the eating elicited by adrenergic stimulation of the paraventricular nucleus, Brain Research (1981) 225,(2):249-269
540. Cani PD, Amar J, Iglesias MA, Poggi M, Knauf C, Bastelica D, Neyrinck AM, Fava F, Tuohy KM, Chabo C, Waget A, Delmée E, Cousin B, Sulpice T, Chamontin B, Ferrières J, Tanti JF, Gibson GR, Casteilla L, Delzenne NM, Alessi MC, Burcelin R. Metabolic endotoxemia initiates obesity and insulin resistance. Diabetes. 2007;56,7,1761-72.
541. Turnbaugh, P.J., Ley, R.E., Mahowald, M.A., Magrini, V., Mardis, E.R., and Gordon, J.I. "An obesity-associated gut microbiome with increased capacity for energy harvest". 2006;Nature 444, 1027–1031

References

542. Rook G A.W. Regulation of the immune system by biodiversity from the natural environment: An ecosystem service essential to health P Natl Acad Sci (2013);110:18360–7.
543. A J. Prussin, II and L C. Marr. Sources of airborne microorganisms in the built environment. Microbiome. (2015); 3: 78.
544. Devkota S, Wang Y, Musch MW, Leone V, Fehlner-Peach H, Nadimpalli A, Antonopoulos DA, Jabri B, Chang EB. Dietary-fat-induced taurocholic acid promotes pathobiont expansion and colitis in Il10-/- mice. Nature. (2012);487(7405):104-8.
545. Dominguez-Bello MG, Costello EK, Contreras M, et al. Delivery mode shapes the acquisition and structure of the initial microbiota across multiple body habitats in newborns. *Proceedings of the National Academy of Sciences of the United States of America*. 2010;107(26): 11971-11975.
546. Lips P. Worldwide status of vitamin D nutrition. J Steroid Biochem Mol Biol. (2010);121(1-2):297-300.
547. Gordon CM, DePeter KC, Feldman HA, Grace E, Emans SJ. Prevalence of vitamin D deficiency among healthy adolescents. Arch Pediatr Adolesc Med. (2004);158(6):531-7.
548. Holick MF. Vitamin D deficiency. N Engl J Med. (2007) 19;357(3): 266-81.
549. Forney LA, Earnest CP, Henagan TM, Johnson LE, Castleberry TJ, Stewart LK. Vitamin D status, body composition, and fitness measures in college-aged students. J Strength Cond Res. (2014);28(3):814-24.
550. Vitezova A, Muka T, Zillikens MC, Voortman T, Uitterlinden AG, Hofman A, Rivadeneira F, Kiefte-de Jong JC, Franco OH. Vitamin D and body composition in the elderly. Clin Nutr. (2017);36(2):585-592.
551. LH Foo, Q Zhang, K Zhu, G Ma, A Trube, H Greenfield, DR Fraser. Relationship between vitamin D status, body composition and physical exercise of adolescent girls in Beijing. Osteoporosis International (2009); 20 (3):417-425
552. Earthman CP, Beckman LM, Masodkar K, Sibley SD. The link between obesity and low circulating 25-hydroxyvitamin D concentrations: considerations and implications. Int J Obes (Lond). 2012 Mar;36(3): 387-96.
553. Hossein-nezhad A, Spira A, Holick MF. Influence of Vitamin D Status and Vitamin D3 Supplementation on Genome Wide Expression of White Blood Cells: A Randomized Double-Blind Clinical Trial" PLoS ONE (2013) 8(3): e58725.

References

554. Bikle DD. Vitamin D regulation of immune function. Vitam Horm. 2011;86:1-21.
555. Yin L, Grandi N, Raum E, Haug U, Arndt V, Brenner H. Meta-analysis: longitudinal studies of serum vitamin D and colorectal cancer risk. *Aliment Pharmacol Ther.* (2009); 30:113-25.
556. McNamee, D. Vitamin D supplements may reverse progression of low-grade prostate tumors. Medical News Today. (2015, March 23)
557. Michalsen A, Li C. Fasting therapy - an expert panel update of the 2002 consensus guidelines. Forsch Komplementmed. (2013);20(6):434-43. doi: 10.1159/000357602.
558. Weindruch R, Walford RL. The retardation of aging and disease by dietary restriction. Springfield, Ill., U.S.A: C.C. Thomas; 1988.
559. McCorry, LK. "Physiology of the autonomic nervous system.". *American journal of pharmaceutical education.* 2007; **71** (4): 78.
560. Halagappa VK, Guo Z, Pearson M, Matsuoka Y, Cutler RG, Laferla FM, Mattson MP. Intermittent fasting and caloric restriction ameliorate age-related behavioral deficits in the triple-transgenic mouse model of Alzheimer's disease. Neurobiology of disease. 2007;26:212–220.
561. Arumugam TV, Phillips TM, Cheng A, Morrell CH, Mattson MP, Wan R. Age and energy intake interact to modify cell stress pathways and stroke outcome. Annals of neurology. 2010;67:41–52.
562. Hartman AL, Rubenstein JE, Kossoff EH. Intermittent fasting: A "new" historical strategy for controlling seizures? *Epilepsy research.* 2013;104(3):275-279. doi:10.1016/j.eplepsyres.2012.10.011.
563. Varady KA, Hellerstein MK. Alternate-day fasting and chronic disease prevention: a review of human and animal trials. Am J Clin Nutr. 2007;86:7–13.
564. Pedersen CR, Hagemann I, Bock T, Buschard K. Intermittent feeding and fasting reduces diabetes incidence in BB rats. Autoimmunity. 1999;30:243–250.
565. Ahmet I, Wan R, Mattson MP, Lakatta EG, Talan M. Cardioprotection by intermittent fasting in rats. Circulation. 2005;112:3115–3121.
566. Castello L, Froio T, Maina M, Cavallini G, Biasi F, Leonarduzzi G, Donati A, Bergamini E, Poli G, Chiarpotto E. Alternate-day fasting protects the rat heart against age-induced inflammation and fibrosis by inhibiting oxidative damage and NF-kB activation. Free Radic Biol Med. 2010;48:47–54.
567. Remely M, Hippe B, Geretschlaeger I, Stegmayer S, Hoefinger I, Haslberger A. Increased gut microbiota diversity and abundance of

References

Faecalibacterium prausnitzii and Akkermansia after fasting: a pilot study. Wien Klin Wochenschr. 2015 May;127(9-10):394-8.

568. Dolinoy DC, Huang D, Jirtle RL. "Maternal nutrient supplementation counteracts bisphenol A-induced DNA hypomethylation in early development", PNAS 104: 13056–13061. (2007) PMID 17670942

569. Huang EJ, Reichardt LF. "Neurotrophins: Roles in Neuronal Development and Function". Annu. Rev. Neurosci; 2001; 24, 677–736. doi:10.1146/annurev.neuro.24.1.677. PMC 2758233. PMID 11520916

570. Fu L, Doreswamy V, Prakash R. "The biochemical pathways of central nervous system neural degeneration in niacin deficiency". Neural Regen Res; 2014; 9,16, 1509–1513. doi:10.4103/1673-5374.139475. PMC 4192966. PMID 25317166

571. Heinonen I, Kalliokoski KK, Hannukainen JC, Duncker DJ, Nuutila P, Knuuti J. Organ-Specific Physiological Responses to Acute Physical Exercise and Long-Term Training in Humans. Physiology (Bethesda); 2014;29,6, 421–436. doi:10.1152/physiol.00067.2013. PMID 25362636

572. Perrey S. Promoting Motor Function by Exercising the Brain. Brain Sciences. 2013;3,1,101-122. doi:10.3390/brainsci3010101.

573. Phillips C, Baktir MA, Srivatsan M, Salehi A. "Neuroprotective effects of physical activity on the brain: a closer look at trophic factor signaling". Front Cell Neurosci; 2014; 8, 170. doi:10.3389/fncel.2014.00170. PMC 4064707. PMID 24999318

574. Denham J, Marques FZ, O'Brien BJ, Charchar FJ. Exercise: putting action into our epigenome. Sports Med; 2014; 44, 2, 189–209. doi: 10.1007/s40279-013-0114-1. PMID

575. Teresa T Fung, Vasanti Malik, Kathryn M Rexrode, JoAnn E Manson, Walter C Willett, and Frank B Hu. Sweetened beverage consumption and risk of coronary heart disease in women. Am J Clin Nutr; 2009; 89 ,4, 1037-1042

576. LaMonte MJ, Blair SN. Physical activity, cardiorespiratory fitness, and adiposity: contributions to disease risk. Curr Opin Clin Nutr Metab Care; 2006 Sep ;9(5):540-6.

577. Johnson MS, Figueroa-Colon R, Herd SL, Fields DA, Sun M, Hunter GR, Goran MI. Aerobic fitness, not energy expenditure, influences subsequent increase in adiposity in black and white children. Pediatrics; 2000; 106(4):E50.

578. Blair SN, Brodney S. Effects of physical inactivity and obesity on morbidity and mortality: current evidence and research issues. Med Sci Sports Exerc; 1999; 31(11 Suppl):S646-62.

References

579. Russo GL. Dietary n-6 and n-3 polyunsaturated fatty acids: from biochemistry to clinical implications in cardiovascular prevention. Biochem Pharmacol; 2009; 15;77,6, 937-46. doi: 10.1016/j.bcp.2008.10.020.
580. A.P. Simopoulos. Evolutionary aspects of diet, the omega-6/omega-3 ratio and genetic variation: nutritional implications for chronic diseases. Biomedicine & Pharmacotherapy; 2006 ;60, 9, Pages 502-507
581. A Jenkinson, M F Franklin, K Wahle, G G Duthie. Dietary intakes of polyunsaturated fatty acids and indices of oxidative stress in human volunteers; Eur J Clin Nutr; 1999; 53, 7, 523-528.
582. David JA Jenkins, Cyril WC Kendall, Livia SA Augustin, Silvia Franceschi, Maryam Hamidi, Augustine Marchie, Alexandra L Jenkins, and Mette Axelsen. Glycemic index: overview of implications in health and disease. Am J Clin Nutr; 2002; 76 ,1 , 266S-273S.
583. Frank B Hu. Are refined carbohydrates worse than saturated fat? Am J Clin Nutr; 2010; 91, 6 ,1541-1542
584. David S. Ludwig, MD, PhD, Joseph A. Majzoub, MD, Ahmad Al-Zahrani, M*, Gerard E. Dallal, PhD, Isaac Blanco, Susan B. Roberts, PhD. High Glycemic Index Foods, Overeating, and Obesity. Pediatrics; 1999; 103,3 , pp. e26 (doi: 10.1542/peds.103.3.e26)
585. Stanhope KL, Schwarz JM, Havel PJ. Adverse metabolic effects of dietary fructose: results from the recent epidemiological, clinical, and mechanistic studies. Curr Opin Lipidol. 2013;24,3:198-206. doi: 10.1097/MOL.0b013e3283613bca.
586. Heather Basciano, Lisa Federico and Khosrow Adeli. Fructose, insulin resistance, and metabolic dyslipidemia. Nutrition & Metabolism. 2005; 2:5 doi:10.1186/1743-7075-2-5
587. Kimber L. Stanhope, Jean Marc Schwarz, Nancy L. Keim, Steven C. Griffen, Andrew A. Bremer, James L. Graham, Bonnie Hatcher, Chad L. Cox, Artem Dyachenko, Wei Zhang, John P. McGahan, Anthony Seibert, Ronald M. Krauss, Sally Chiu, Ernst J. Schaefer, Masumi Ai, Seiko Otokozawa, Katsuyuki Nakajima, Takamitsu Nakano, Carine Beysen, Marc K. Hellerstein, Lars Berglund,and Peter J. Havel. Consuming fructose-sweetened, not glucose-sweetened, beverages increases visceral adiposity and lipids and decreases insulin sensitivity in overweight/obese humans. J Clin Invest. 2009; 119,5: 1322–1334. doi: 10.1172/JCI37385
588. Schulze MB, Manson JE, Ludwig DS, et al. Sugar-Sweetened Beverages, Weight Gain, and Incidence of Type 2 Diabetes in Young

References

and Middle-Aged Women. JAMA. 2004;292(8):927-934. doi:10.1001/jama.292.8.927.

589. Basu S, Yoffe P, Hills N, Lustig RH. The Relationship of Sugar to Population-Level Diabetes Prevalence: An Econometric Analysis of Repeated Cross- Sectional Data. PLoS ONE. 2013;8,2: e57873. doi: 10.1371/journal.pone.0057873

590. Ludwig, David S et al. Relation between consumption of sugar-sweetened drinks and childhood obesity: a prospective, observational analysis. The Lancet. 2001; 357, 9255, 505 - 508

591. Richard J Johnson, Mark S Segal, Yuri Sautin, Takahiko Nakagawa, Daniel I Feig, Duk-Hee Kang, Michael S Gersch, Steven Benner, and Laura G Sánchez-Lozada. Potential role of sugar (fructose) in the epidemic of hypertension, obesity and the metabolic syndrome, diabetes, kidney disease, and cardiovascular disease. Am J Clin Nutr. 2007;86,4 899-906

592. Seely, StephenHorrobin, David F et al. Diet and breast cancer: The possible connection with sugar consumption. Medical Hypotheses. 1983. 11, 3:319 - 327 DOI: http://dx.doi.org/10.1016/0306-9877(83)90095-6

593. Strazzullo, Pasquale; D'Elia, Lanfranco; Kandala, Ngianga-Bakwin; Cappuccio, Francesco P. "Salt intake, stroke, and cardiovascular disease: meta-analysis of prospective studies". British Medical Journal; 2009; 339 (b4567). doi:10.1136/bmj.b4567. PMC 2782060. PMID 19934192.

594. Garg R, Williams GH, Hurwitz S, Brown NJ, Hopkins PN, Adler GK. Low Salt Diet Increases Insulin Resistance in Healthy Subjects. Metabolism: clinical and experimental; 2011;60,7, 965-968. doi: 10.1016/j.metabol.2010.09.005.

595. Barnard RJ, Gonzalez JH, Liva ME, Ngo TH. Effects of a low-fat, high-fiber diet and exercise program on breast cancer risk factors in vivo and tumor cell growth and apoptosis in vitro. Nutr Cancer. 2006;55(1): 28-34.

596. Soliman S, Aronson WJ, Barnard RJ. Analyzing Serum-Stimulated Prostate Cancer Cell Lines After Low-Fat, High-Fiber Diet and Exercise Intervention. Evid Based Complement Alternat Med; 2009; Volume 2011, 1-7. Article ID 529053 doi:10.1093/ecam/nep031

597. Boffetta, P., Couto, E., Wichmann, J., et al. Fruit and vegetable intake and overall cancer risk in the European prospective investigation into cancer (EPIC). J. Natl. Cancer Inst; 2010; 102,8, 529–537.

References

598. Rashmi Sinha; Amanda J. Cross; Barry I. Graubard; Michael F. Leitzmann; Arthur Schatzkin. Meat Intake and Mortality: A Prospective Study of Over Half a Million People. Arch Intern Med; 2009;169,6,:562-571.
599. Ngo TH, Barnard RJ, Tymchuk CN, Cohen P, Aronson. Effect of diet and exercise on serum insulin, IGF-I, and IGFBP-1 levels and growth of LNCaP cells in vitro (United States). Cancer Causes Control; 2002;13,10,929-35.
600. McCarty MF. Vegan proteins may reduce risk of cancer, obesity, and cardiovascular disease by promoting increased glucagon activity. Med Hypotheses; 1999;53,6,459-85.
601. Boffetta, P., Couto, E., Wichmann, J., et al. Fruit and vegetable intake and overall cancer risk in the European prospective investigation into cancer (EPIC). J. Natl. Cancer Inst; 2010; 102,8, 529–537.
602. Donkena, K.V., Young, C.Y.F., and Tindall, D.J. Oxidative stress and DNA methylation in prostate cancer. Obstetrics and Gynecology Intl; 2010; Article ID 302051. doi:10.1155/2010/302051.
603. Duessel, S., Heuertz, R.M, and Ezekiel, U.R. Growth inhibition of human colon cancer cells by plant compounds. Clin. Lab. Sci; 2008; 21,3, 151–157.
604. Fang, M., Chen, D., and Yang, C.S. Dietary polyphenols may affect DNA methylation. J. Nutr; 2007; 137: 223S–228S.
605. Hung, H.-C., Joshipura, K.J., Jiang, R., et al. Fruit and vegetable intake and risk of major chronic disease. J. Natl. Cancer Inst; 2004; 96,21, 1577–1584.
606. Jump DB, Tripathy S, Depner CM. (2013) Fatty acid-regulated transcription factors in the liver. Annu Rev Nutr; 2013; 33,249-269.
607. Shanmugam MK, Sethi G. Role of epigenetics in inflammation-associated diseases. Subcell Biochem; 2013;61,627-57. doi: 10.1007/978-94-007-4525-4_27.
608. McIntosh M, Miller C. A diet containing food rich in soluble and insoluble fiber improves glycemic control and reduces hyperlipidemia among patients with type 2 diabetes mellitus. Nutr Rev; 2001;59,2,52-5.
609. Ensminger AH, Esminger M. K. J. e. al. Food for Health: A Nutrition Encyclopedia. Clovis, California: Pegus Press. (1986). PMID:15210.
610. Wood, Rebecca. The Whole Foods Encyclopaedia. New York, NY: Prentice-Hall Press. (1988). PMID:15220.
611. Alexander DD, Weed DL, Cushing CA, Lowe KA. Meta-analysis of prospective studies of red meat consumption and colorectal cancer. Eur

References

J Cancer Prev. 2011 Jul;20(4)293-307. doi: 10.1097/CEJ 0b013e328345f985.

612. Xinmin S. Li, Slayman Obeid, Roland Klingenberg, Baris Gencer, François Mach, Lorenz Räber, Stephan Windecker, Nicolas Rodondi, David Nanchen, Olivier Muller, Melroy X. Miranda, Christian M. Matter, Yuping Wu, Lin Li, Zeneng Wang, Hassan S. Alamri, Valentin Gogonea, Yoon-Mi Chung, W.H. Wilson Tang, Stanley L. Hazen, Thomas F. Lüscher; Gut microbiome-dependent trimethylamine N-oxide in acute coronary syndromes: a prognostic marker for incident cardiovascular events beyond traditional risk factors. *Eur Heart J* 2017 ehw582. doi: 10.1093/eurheartj/ehw582

613. Stanhope KL, Schwarz JM, Havel PJ. Adverse metabolic effects of dietary fructose: results from the recent epidemiological, clinical, and mechanistic studies. Curr Opin Lipidol; 2013 Jun;24(3):198-206. doi: 10.1097/MOL.0b013e3283613bca.

614. George A Bray, Samara Joy Nielsen, and Barry M Popkin. Consumption of high-fructose corn syrup in beverages may play a role in the epidemic of obesity. Am J Clin Nutr; 2004;79, 4 , 537-543.

615. Basu S, Yoffe P, Hills N, Lustig RH. The Relationship of Sugar to Population-Level Diabetes Prevalence: An Econometric Analysis of Repeated Cross- Sectional Data.

616. Basu S, Yoffe P, Hills N, Lustig RH. The relationship of sugar to population-level diabetes prevalence: an econometric analysis of repeated cross-sectional data. PLoS One. 2013;8(2):e57873. doi: 10.1371/journal.pone.0057873.

617. Teresa T Fung, Vasanti Malik, Kathryn M Rexrode, JoAnn E Manson, Walter C Willett, and Frank B Hu. Sweetened beverage consumption and risk of coronary heart disease in women. Am J Clin Nutr; 2009; 89 ,4, 1037-1042

618. T Norat et al. Meat, fish, and colorectal cancer risk: the European prospective investigation into cancer and nutrition. Journal of the National Cancer Institute 2005 97: 906-916

619. Chao A, Thun MJ, Connell CJ, McCullough ML, Jacobs EJ, Flanders WD, Rodriguez C, Sinha R, Calle EE. Meat consumption and risk of colorectal cancer. JAMA. 2005; 12;293(2):172-82.

620. Wollowski I, Rechkemmer G, Pool-Zobel BL. Protective role of probiotics and prebiotics in colon cancer. Am J Clin Nutr. 2001;73:451S-455S. PMID: 11157356

References

All Books By Galit Goldfarb

1. The Guerrilla Diet & Lifestyle Program - Wage War On Weight and Poor Health and Learn To Thrive In The Modern Jungle.
2. How to Achieve Success and Happiness series:

    1. The 6 Principle Strategy for Creating a Successful & Happy Life: Book # 1: The Basics Everyone Needs to Know
    2. The 6 Principle Strategy for Creating a Successful & Happy Life: Book # 2: How to Create Peace of Mind
    3. The 6 Principle Strategy for Creating a Successful & Happy Life: Book # 3: How to Create Optimum Health
    4. The 6 Principle Strategy for Creating a Successful & Happy Life: Book # 4: How to Create Great Relationships
    5. The 6 Principle Strategy for Creating a Successful & Happy Life: Book # 5: How to Create Wealth

3. Best Way To Lose Weight - A Step-By-Step Guide to Lose Weight In A Month The Guerrilla Diet Way
4. 50 Best Recipes For Health and Weight Loss - The Guerrilla Diet Way

Chapter 14 - The Guerrilla Diet Shopping List

5.

Printed in Great Britain
by Amazon